Building the Reflective Healthcare Organisation

Building the Reflective Healthcare Organisation

Tony Ghaye

Director, The International Institute of Reflective Practice-UK
and
Visiting Professor at Luleå University of Technology, Sweden

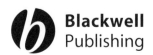

Blackwell
Publishing

Blackwell Publishing editorial offices:
Blackwell Publishing Ltd, 9600 Garsington Road, Oxford OX4 2DQ, UK
Tel: +44 (0)1865 776868
Blackwell Publishing Inc., 350 Main Street, Malden MA 02148-5020, USA
Tel: +1 781 388 8250
Blackwell Publishing Asia Pty Ltd, 550 Swanston Street, Carlton, Victoria 3053, Australia
Tel: +61 (0)3 8359 1011

First published 2008 by Blackwell Publishing Ltd

ISBN-13: 978-1-4051-0589-7

Library of Congress Cataloging-in-Publication Data

Ghaye, Tony.
    Building the reflective healthcare organisation / Tony Ghaye.
        p. ; cm.
    Includes bibliographical references and index.
    ISBN-13: 978-1-4051-0589-7 (pbk. : alk. paper)
 1. Health services administration.
 2. Reflective teaching. 3. Organizational change. I. Title.
        [DNLM: 1. Health Services Administration. 2. Organizational Innovation.
 3. Problem-Based Learning—methods. W 84 G411b 2007]
    RA971.G48 2007
    362.1068—dc22   2007008606

A catalogue record for this title is available from the British Library

Set in 10/12.5 Palatino
by Charontec Ltd (A Macmillan Company), Chennai, India
Printed and bound in Singapore
by Utopia Press Pte Ltd

The publisher's policy is to use permanent paper from mills that operate a sustainable forestry policy, and which has been manufactured from pulp processed using acid-free and elementary chlorine-free practices. Furthermore, the publisher ensures that the text paper and cover board used have met acceptable environmental accreditation standards.

For further information on Blackwell Publishing, visit our website:
www.blackwellnursing.com

Contents

Acknowledgements

I would like to thank all those who, by their special gifts and talents, have enabled me to write this book.

First and foremost I'd like to thank all the staff and users of healthcare services who have contributed to the ideas in this book, in so many ways. Through wonderfully uplifting and challenging conversations, I have come to a much deeper appreciation of what it is you care about deeply and passionately. You know who you are. I hope you feel your spirit within the covers of this book. A special acknowledgement is given to Jane Marr. Thank you for having confidence in me and reflective learning.

I owe a very special debt of gratitude to two colleagues from Luleå University of Technology, who have not only been wonderful coffee-drinking company but who have also added so much depth to my thinking about working appreciatively with others: they are Anita Melander-Wikman, Department of Health Sciences, and Maria Jansson, Department of Business Administration and Social Sciences.

Several colleagues from the editorial board of the international peer-reviewed journal *Reflective Practice* have read drafts of each action step, made suggestions and provided information and insight. I thank them all. My special thanks are extended to Sue Lillyman for her considerable support over the years and belief in the goodness that comes from reflective learning. You have established a link between cream cakes and creativity.

My colleague Karen Deeny has been a source of support and creativity. Many ideas have been hatched during our conversations on Great Western rail journeys from Gloucester to London. Thank you for your open listening to my half-baked ideas and for the skilful way you put appreciative intelligence into practice. Also thank you for your 'lists' of discussion topics and jobs to do.

Without the excellent administrative skills of Jules Holland, the senior administrative officer of the Institute of Reflective Practice-UK, bringing this book to fruition would have been so much harder. Thank you for your attention to detail and wonderful ICT skills. Sincere thanks also go to Sue Hampton for the conscientious way she completed the grunge jobs in her usual cheerful way.

Finally, I could not have asked for a better team of staff to bring this book to fruition than Beth Knight and Katharine Unwin at Blackwell Publishing. Thank you for being so patient with me and for encouraging me in the writing of this book.

Dedication

This book is dedicated to my colleagues and friends in three places: those in the 'arctic north' and working to improve the psychosocial well-being of children there; and those working for EASUN and undertaking groundbreaking work through grassroots strengthening and capacity building in East Africa. I also dedicate this book to those in the Research Unit of the College of Social Work of the University of Mumbai and those in the Family Service Centre. I acknowledge and appreciate the great work you are doing in the slum community of Ambedkar Nagar in South Mumbai. The way in which you address the scale, urgency and complexity of child-protection issues there, so that children can lead happy and fulfilling lives, is inspirational.

Preface

Which way is this book heading? In the direction of a kind of workplace I'm calling 'the reflective healthcare organisation'.

> . . . of course the future is hard to see. But we're all heading that way anyhow, and as difficult as it may be to envision, we have to make some decisions about which futures to aim for and which to avoid.

(Gilbert 2006, pp. 212–13)

To get there from where we are now, we have to scale up the practices of reflection so that they become an organisation-wide good work habit. The evidence I present in this book seems to suggest strongly that this is a worthy thing to do. But ultimately, the benefits of scaling up the practices of reflection must be felt at the point of care. There is still much work to be done to bridge the gaps between reflective practices that benefit healthcare professionals and those that benefit clients and patients. Although we still have much to do and learn, we appear to be moving in a positive direction. But it is not a simple task. This is not only because of the sheer complexity of healthcare systems, mounting financial pressures and increasing demand for better value for money. It is also because, right now, we are by no means good at scaling up reflection. There are obstacles to overcome and challenges to be met. But most important of all is the need to change the way we think about obstacles and challenges (Seddon 2006). We need to change our obsession with problems, because this is often the problem. If the situation is difficult to change, then we may have to alter the way we think about it. We may have to try to see or frame things differently, to create new realities by interacting in new ways. Creative interactions, appreciative conversations and supportive relationships are some of the characteristics of the reflective organisation. With these, things get better. If patterns of interaction remain the same, or get worse, ground is lost (Fullan 2001). It is unwise to think that in a target-driven UK National Health Service (NHS) we can do things the way we've always done them and yet expect different results.

This book may therefore require you to make a significant shift in your thinking and in your relationships with others. It may necessitate leaving a paradigm (a collection of values, ideas, processes and outcomes) that may be familiar and comfortable. The current dominant western worldview espouses individualism, autonomy, independence and progress through problem-solving (Stavros and Torres 2005). This book is about reframing this. *Building the Reflective Healthcare Organisation* is a call to change the way we normally view our work and interactions with others.

Many healthcare organisations are trying to do just this. Evidence of it comes in the form of flatter structures, more dynamic systems thinking, attention being given to creating healthy working relationships and calls for leadership at every level. This book is about building and sustaining a reflective organisation by acting with appreciative intent.

> **Invitation**
> To think about the idea of a reflective organisation

So where does this book begin? By acknowledging that most people practise reflection alone. This bias towards reflection as an individualistic practice means that any benefits accrue to individuals and not to the organisation. Any reflective learning (r-learning) that arises is specific to the context in which individuals are working – and we know that there are limits to learning alone. This individualistic practice is important but not sufficient for building a reflective organisation. An erroneous assumption is that if we produce enough individual reflective practitioners, then somehow we build a reflective organisation. This is questionable, because such an organisation is based on a culture of collectivism, not individualism, on collective learning processes, not individual practices. These collective processes need to be embedded within workgroups to enable them to develop into reflective healthcare teams (Ghaye 2005). When we talk of reflective teams, we have significantly scaled up r-learning. It is reflection on a bigger scale. This is where people are learning with others and building a collective wisdom. I cannot stress enough the critical importance of organising for, and systematically learning from, each other and how this contributes to building the reflective organisation.

> **Invitation**
> To think about how to scale up reflection

In this book I try to take the mystery, but not the complexity, out of building a reflective healthcare organisation. I combine two metaphors to help me respond to the book's central question:

> How can we scale up reflective learning so that it becomes a collegial and useful, organisation-wide, sustainable work habit?

The metaphors I use throughout the book are those of 'a journey' (Van de Ven *et al.* 1999) over 'rough ground' (Blair 2006). I begin this journey by trying to develop an appreciation in your mind of the range of conceptions, variety of practices and a flavour of the internal debates currently associated with the term 'reflective practice'. From my analysis of contemporary work in the field emerges a positive re-framing of reflective practice as r-learning. I then go on to describe four basic intentions of r-learning that support and can sustain the reflective organisation. These r-learning intentions are to:

- develop an appreciation of other's feelings, thoughts and quality of action;
- re-frame experience so that we can better understand our conviction-laden practices and create new and improved realities;
- build a collective wisdom through conversations of positive regard;
- achieve and move forward by seeing how the future unfolds from the present.

Invitation
To think about the intentions of r-learning

The book then points towards some action *pathways-to-scale*. Each one helps us make progress towards a reflective organisation. I set out six of them:

- *Values pathway*, where we develop a congruence between our espoused values and our values-in-action.
- *Conversation pathway*, which involves using the power of the positive question.
- *User pathway*, where we learn from patient and client experiences.
- *Leadership pathway*, where leaders use their appreciative intelligence.
- *Team pathway*, where knowledge is created and learning is shared within and between teams.
- *Network pathway*, where linked groups/teams work in a knowledge-sharing way.

Invitation
To think about the notion of pathways-to-scale

So we have a vision, four intentions and some pathways-to-scale. The only thing missing is a *force for change* – something that energises and fuels the whole enterprise. That gets us 'there' from where we are now. RAISE is one such force for change that enables us to scale up r-learning. I call the five related forces:

R = reflecting
A = appreciating
I = interacting
S = strategising
E = energising.

Why do our brains stubbornly insist on projecting us into the future when there is so much to think about right here today? The most obvious answer to that question is that thinking about the future can be pleasurable ... when people daydream about the future; they tend to imagine themselves achieving and succeeding rather than fumbling or failing. Indeed, thinking about the future can be so pleasurable that sometimes we'd rather think about it than get there.

(Gilbert 2006, pp. 16–17)

So from this point onwards, you are provided with an opportunity to think through how you might begin to build a reflective healthcare organisation.

References

Blair, D. (2006) *Wittgenstein, Language and Information: 'Back to the Rough Ground!'*. Springer-Verlag, New York.

Fullan, M. (2001) *Leading in a Culture of Change*. Jossey-Bass, San Francisco, CA.

Ghaye, T. (2005) *Developing the Reflective Healthcare Team*. Blackwell Publishing, Oxford.

Gilbert, D. (2006) *Stumbling on Happiness*. HarperCollins, London.

Seddon, J. (2006) Beware 'tool heads' bearing targets – they won't make things any better for the patient. *Health Services Journal*, 7 September, 23.

Stavros, J.M. & Torres, C.B. (2005) *Dynamic Relationships: Unleashing the Power of Appreciative Inquiry in Daily Living*. Taos Institute Publications, Chagrin Falls, OH.

Van de Ven, A.H., Polley, D., Garud, R. & Venkataraman. S. (1999) *The Innovation Journey*. Oxford University Press, New York and Oxford.

Introduction: mapping out the 'rough ground'

The aim of this book is to give you an overview of a kind of organisation, fully fit for purpose and adaptable, that is suited to a world of rapid and complex changes in healthcare. I call it the reflective organisation. For many years, energy and resources have been devoted to the education of reflective practitioners. More recently, with much healthcare reform depending on groups of staff working together and in different ways, there has been an increasing focus on developing reflective healthcare teams.

This book goes one step further and describes the attributes and work habits of an emerging form of organisation, a reflective organisation. Put simply, such an organisation links the power of asking the positive question with positive action. It describes how these are fuelled by the process of reflective learning. *Building the Reflective Healthcare Organisation* is not a cookbook or blueprint. It is a thinking guide to develop services, improve patient/client experiences and enrich working life. It is, therefore, a book of hope and optimism. To help you think through the applications and implications of the contents of the book for your own organisation, I use two metaphors. The first is Van de Ven *et al.*'s (1999) notion of a 'journey'. The second is Wittgenstein's idea of 'rough ground' (Blair 2006).

Additionally, to help you navigate your way through this book, I introduce action steps 1, 2 and 3 in two ways.

- by summarising the big ideas the step contains as a collection of 'ideas bundles';
- by linking the ideas bundles together in the form of a 'mind map' (Buzan 2006).

For example, this introduction contains six major *ideas bundles*, which provide direction for building a reflective healthcare organisation. They are:

Bundle 1 **The positive core**
This is a book about using the power of the positive question, positive action and reflective learning. It thinks through a response to the following question: How can we scale up reflective learning so that it becomes a collegial and useful, organisation-wide, sustainable work habit?

Bundle 2 **(Re-)framing reflective practice**
This book re-frames reflective practice as reflective learning. It suggests that we need to re-see some customary ways of thinking about reflection – to think of it more as a political and collective process and not only as a professional and individualistic practice.

Bundle 3   **R-learning**
This stands for reflective learning. It has four principle intentions. I also suggest that this learning can be characterised in four ways as being appreciative, generative, transcending and transformative.

Bundle 4   **Positive action**
After this introduction, the rest of the book is organised into four funda- mental action steps. It sets out six possible action pathways-to-scale. Progress along each pathway is described as a 'journey', one of the two metaphors used in this book.

Bundle 5   **Scaling up**
This book offers a way of scaling up reflective learning, from the individ- ual to an organisation-wide work habit. Much depends upon the way the case is made for this and how staff meet the challenges of taking up such action.

Bundle 6   **Mapping the rough ground**
The experience of building the reflective healthcare organisation may not be one of working in Schön's swampy lowlands or on the high ground. In this book I suggest that the experiential journey is more like traversing *rough ground*. This is the second metaphor used in the book.

So how do these six *ideas bundles* link up to form a coherent and under- standable introduction? Fig. 0.1 shows this.

Building the reflective healthcare organisation: asking a question

How do we frame the challenge of building the reflective healthcare organisation as a question rather than as a problem?

Asking questions that matter can be difficult because we are so used to thinking in terms of problems – root causes of problems to be discovered, problems to be solved, things to be 'fixed'. Sometimes, creative and funda- mental changes can begin when we start to ask questions and to do this together. Asking questions marks the start of a learning conversation. This is a very different experience from many of our normal conversations, which often tend to be about problems. Here, our talking and listening often fail to solve a problem because of the way that most of us talk and listen, most of the time. You may find it hard to accept, but our most com- mon way of talking is telling, asserting this or that, and talking at the expense of asking. Our most common way of listening is not really listen- ing at all. At best, it's an impoverished view of listening, one where we lis- ten only to our own voice, not to the voices of others. If we are unable to talk openly about the complex problems (or challenges) that face us in health service reform, then we get stuck. Also, managing and delivering high-quality health services, to all, in an efficient, cost-effective way is jeopardised if we are unable to listen. So what happens next? There are

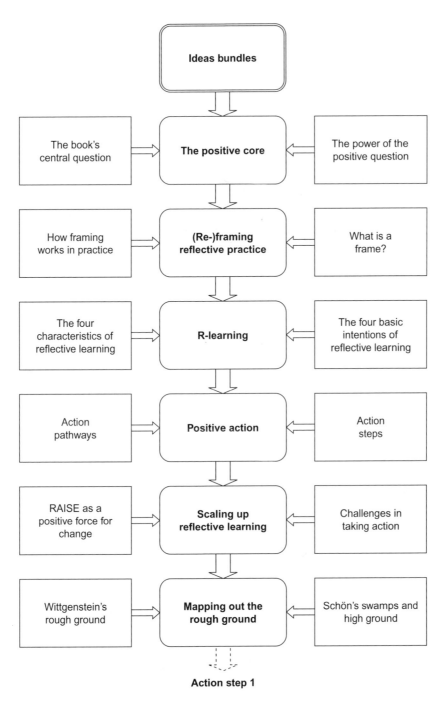

Figure 0.1 A mind map for the introduction: mapping out the rough ground.

two ways to unstick a conversation. The first is for one person or group to act unilaterally – to impose on others their solution to the problem by force, by a clever manipulation of a meeting's agenda, use of meeting time, and so on. Another way to get unstuck is to ask a question.

The power of the positive question

There are many kinds of question. The two most common kinds that we ask are open and closed questions. An open question is an invitation to express a point of view. A closed question usually invites a 'yes' or 'no' response. Another kind of question is a *genuine* question – a question for which we don't already have an answer. Genuine questions are an invitation to be creative. They invite new ideas and insight. For example, two district nurses were visiting an elderly woman who had fallen while she was out shopping. She had twisted her ankle badly and bumped her head. The elderly woman couldn't remember much about the incident. One of the nurses suggested to the woman that she stayed at home, rested her leg and didn't think of going to the shops again for a while. The woman became visibly distressed. She enjoyed going to the shops. She wanted to visit the town library and her friends and go to church. The other nurse said: 'What would happen if we thought about this differently?' This carefully framed question, genuine and sincere, invited a new way of understanding the woman's situation. It invited a new and different conversation with her.

A 25-year-old man took a day off work. He went for a cycle ride. He came down a hill, on a narrow lane, at speed. Round a bend he hit a car, coming up the hill the other way. He flew over the length of the car and landed on the lane behind. Staff at a local district general hospital did their best for him. They gave him a CT scan, fixed his broken leg and stitched him up. Thirty-six hours later, just before his discharge, the man complained of a pain in his chest and back. When reviewing his case, the doctor said to the multidisciplinary team: 'What questions have we forgotten to ask that, if we did ask, might make this patient's condition better?' Again, this carefully framed question immediately opened up possibilities for improving the current situation. Clearly, asking questions matters.

Also we have *positive questions*. When we focus on problems, this can so easily *be* the problem. By this, I mean that when we start to enquire into our problems, we begin to construct a world in which problems are central. They become the dominant realities that burden us every day. To ask questions about our failings is to create a world in which failing is focal. Deficit-based questions lead to deficit-based conversations, which in turn lead to deficit-based patterns of action. Yet we can flip this over and apply the same logic more positively. By asking ourselves positive questions, we may bring forth future action of far greater promise. Positive questions invite positive action.

So, what question lies at the heart of this book? What is the question that matters? It is this:

How can we scale up reflective learning so that it becomes a collegial and useful, organisation-wide, sustainable work habit?

Although there will be different readings of this question, I suggest that it implies positive action and reflective learning, both working supportively of each other. This book is an opportunity to *think through* some responses to this question.

Opening up the book's central question

At present, many people who work in healthcare claim to be reflective practitioners. Many reflect thoughtfully on their work. Many do this as a silent, private or solitary activity, when they can. In some organisations, reflective practice is supported by some kind of one-to-one (clinical) supervision or mentoring arrangement. This kind of reflection is usually referred to as self-reflection. It is very much encouraged by the UK's Nursing and Midwifery Council (NMC) in this way:

Clinical supervision should be available to registrants throughout their careers so they can constantly evaluate and improve their contribution to patient/client care. Along with the NMC's PREP (continuing professional development) standard, clinical supervision is an important part of clinical governance. It directly relates to registered nurses. Midwives have their own statutory system of local supervision. The NMC supports the principle of clinical supervision . . . [and] has defined a set of principles, which we believe should underpin any system of clinical supervision that is used. Two of the principles are:

1   Clinical supervision supports practice, enabling registrants to maintain and improve standards of care.
2   Clinical supervision is a practice-focused professional relationship, involving a practitioner reflecting on practice guided by a skilled supervisor . . .

(Nursing and Midwifery Council 2006)

Things are changing

The emphasis is upon individuals reflecting on their work, at some opportune moment, after the event. Many education and training modules, courses and programmes serve to both develop and reinforce this individualistic practice. Having said this, more collegial forms of reflecting on practice have emerged over the past few years – but more about this later. So, my central question may sound a bit futuristic, but let me explain.

Things are changing and fast. In this context, Young (2006) argues that we simply *must* find the time to reflect. He says, despite the critics of reflection:

> Those who knock the evidence base and efficacy of reflection, however, should remember that reflection is part of a nurse's legal and professional accountability. It is indisputable that all healthcare professionals owe a duty of care to their patients and must act reasonably, putting the needs of their patients first at all times. To meet this requirement, nurses should be thoughtful and reflective practitioners, should consider the consequences of their actions and must not act hastily or irrationally . . . Given the current emphasis upon clinical governance and quality improvement, in and out of the NHS, it is increasingly common for potential employers to ask for evidence of experiential learning at interview. Ignore reflection at your peril.

(Young 2006, pp. 22–3)

But the pace and complexity of healthcare reform is putting the pervasive notion of the reflective practitioner under pressure. In most health services, these pressures come from within ourselves as we strive to manage and deliver high-quality care. Our personal standards, commitment and interest in our work influence these pressures. They also come from within the organisation for which we work, and particularly as they try to rebuff the damning verdict by the UK's chief medical officer in his report 'Good Doctors, Safer Patients' (Department of Health 2006). The report says:

> Few chief executive officers of health organisations match the depth of fear of missing budgetary and productivity targets with the strength of their passion to improve quality and safety of services for their consumers.

(Department of Health 2006)

In reality, there is much organisational juggling to be done to successfully manage a number of tensioned relationships, for example between:

- higher-quality services at lower cost;
- higher staff performance with lower occupational health problems;
- the need to adopt new working practices in service areas dominated by cultures of disappointment and cynicism;
- increasing capacity while maintaining safe and appropriate practice;
- equity and excellence;
- working smarter while working ethically.

And there are many more.

Some might argue that a focus by chief executives on money and activity is inaccurate and offensive, a perception that arises as a consequence of pressures from the 'centre', from government. We can sense these pressures in the UK government's use of a particular language, such as that embraced in its commitment to a 'patient-led', 'commissioner-delivered service' with 'strong plural, responsive and flexible provision'. This is part of the 'big picture' – a top-down view, if you like.

Top-down and bottom-up action

If we maintain the polarity of top-down and bottom-up for a moment, it is worth putting on the page the views of one frontline nurse. She describes the pressures, collectively, as a culture shift. She says:

> . . . the NHS reforms are changing the landscape of how nurses work, who they work for and who employs them. The reconfiguration of PCTs [primary care trusts], private finance initiatives and schemes such as payment by results mean more nurses are now working for the NHS while not in fact employed by it. Secondly, . . . the demarcation between the public and private sectors is blurring all the time. The walls have definitely come down. The independent sector has become far more integral for training nurses than it once was. Thirdly, there is the sense that, while as a nurse you may be loyal to the NHS, there is no longer any guarantee that the NHS will be loyal back. The latest swathe of redundancies, recruitment freezes and cutbacks, along with what sometimes feels like a constant treadmill of change and bureaucracy has shaken the confidence of many nurses that they had, in effect, a 'job for life' in the NHS.

(Paton 2006, pp. 18–19)

So where does this leave us? I suggest in two places. First, the energy, creativity and power to implement healthcare reforms successfully does not, and cannot, lie with the individual, but with the collective – put simply, with groups of staff and especially with teams. Staff in teams, the *implementers*, are key figures in the reform process. Reflective practitioners, working supportively in reflective workgroups or teams, can be good implementers. I suggest that there are limits to individualism and particularly to learning alone. Seligman (2006) argues that it can slide into meaninglessness. In a fascinating book, he argues:

> . . . as it becomes apparent that individualism produces a tenfold increase in depression, individualism will become a less appealing creed to live by. A second and perhaps more important factor is meaninglessness . . . one necessary condition for meaning is the attachment to something larger than you are. The larger the entity you can attach yourself to, the more meaning you can derive. To the extent that it is now difficult for young people to take seriously their relationship to God, to care about their duties to their country, or to be part of a large and abiding family, meaning in life will be very difficult to find. The self, to put it another way, is a very poor site for meaning.

(Seligman 2006, p. 287)

In the field of reflective practice, this gives us plenty to respond to and engage with. There are a host of explanations as to why, to date, reflective practice has been swamped by individualistic cultures (see p. 44).

Now, and at least for the next decade, we need to take up the challenge and reap the benefits of collective debate and collective action, embracing organisational power, politics and performance in different ways.

Successful healthcare reform is not simply about making policy responsive to service user needs and weaving the two together. It's also about those people involved feeling some deep sense of ownership of these reforms. With this can come creative and supportive behaviours necessary to focus on system improvement. To spread and sustain innovations in health-service delivery and organisation, we need staff that have a systems-thinking mindscape. When working more collectively, in reflective communities, the implementers have a better chance of doing two things. First, making sense of their own practice and working life; second, (re-)connecting and (re-)conceiving the 'system' of which they are a part, in new ways.

Towards systems thinking

In a democracy, every one of us has choices, in every encounter, every day. Fundamentally they are choices about what kind of world we wish to contribute to bring into reality. Kahane (2004) has a view on this:

> The path forward is about becoming more human, not just more clever. It is about transcending our fears of vulnerability, not finding new ways of protecting ourselves. It is about discovering how to act in service of the whole, not just in service of our own interests.

(Kahane 2004, pp. ii–xii)

This has a ring of systems thinking about it. Another way of expressing 'acting in the service of the whole' is Fullan's (2004) phrase, 'systems thinkers in action'. Senge (1990) popularised the notion of systems thinking in bringing about effective change in organisations. More recently, the work of Fullan (2004) brings to our attention the possibility that, despite what Senge claimed, 'We have made no gains in conceptualising, let alone promoting, systems thinking on the ground' (Fullan 2004, p. 8). Fullan believes that little has been done to promote the 'in action' part. Across health and social care, this might be a little harsh. Over the past few years, the NHS Modernisation Agency would argue, I feel, that a number of health and social care communities that, for example, have participated in the Pursuing Perfection initiative led by the Institute for Healthcare Improvement (IHI), are beginning to develop a culture of 'systems' thinking. The more one reads about a focus on looking 'upstream' for solutions to 'problem areas', particularly in the context of improving flow through the system and ensuring that care is provided as close to home as possible, the more this becomes believable. But Fullan's basic point is still worth considering – that what is needed is 'systems thinkers in action' (Fullan 2004, p. 15). Essentially, these are people who can see and promote the interconnectedness of practice. So another question begins to bubble up: How can the scaling-up of learning through the practices of reflection enable healthcare staff to develop a 'literacy of the system'? This, I feel, requires a pretty fundamental shift in professional focus, energy and, above all, mind.

Re-framing reflective practice as reflective learning

The book's central question, in its simplest form, is fundamentally about three things: *practice* (what you and your colleagues do), *place* (where you and your colleagues work) and *learning* (how you and your colleagues learn about yourselves, your work and workplace in order to improve services further, through reflective practices). The conviction-laden value that holds these three together is about achieving and sustaining the best practice possible for the benefit of patients/clients.

There are many kinds of reflection, for example reflection in and on action, anticipatory and retrospective reflection, critical and emancipatory reflection, self-reflection and reflection for improvement. There are also many kinds of practice, for example professional and clinical practice, moral practice, radical practice, ethical and discursive practice and an epistemology of practice (van Manen 1999). There are many kinds of learning, for example experiential and stimulus-response learning, rote and meaningful learning, and deep and surface learning. Then, of course, there is reflective practice and reflective learning. Could our practice ever be anything but reflective? How far can we legitimately talk about unreflective practice? Is this safe, ethical and responsible practice? Could we ever argue convincingly that healthcare professionals should be unreflective in their practice?

What is a frame?

This book re-frames reflective practice as reflective learning – reflective learning done before, during or after an event, alone or with others. It sees reflection as a social practice that focuses on what we do, where, with and for whom. It is thoughtful and considered action, supported by others, that enables us to appreciate what to say and do next. It is learning that provides opportunities for improving what we do. Learning gives us reasons why doing something different might be a good idea. We need to learn from the processes of reflection in order to successfully meet the challenges of healthcare reform. From the work of Dewey (1933) to the present day, many have argued that we learn from past events by working our way through reflective cycles, stages, steps and questions (or 'cues'). Put simply, it is action, and reflection upon it, that can lead to new (and, hopefully, better) actions.

What I have just done is to frame reflective practice in a particular way. It may or may not be a way that you find agreeable. What I have to say in this introduction is that this book requires a radical shift, or re-framing, of our customary ways of thinking about reflective practice – a shift away from the individual and towards the collective, from an apolitical stance to a much more politically literate stance. By 'political', I mean a kind of reflection that embraces a literacy that enables us to read and influence the landscape of change. So let's look at how framing works in practice.

How framing works in practice

Frames have been used in various fields, including healthcare, education, psychology and sociology (Gonos 1997, Johns 2004, Taylor 2000), business management (Goldratt 1990, Watzlawick *et al.* 1974), artificial intelligence (Minsky 1975), decision-making (Kahneman & Tversky 1979), negotiation (Gray 1989, Neale & Bazerman 1985, Pinkley 1990) and environmental conflict management (Lewicki *et al.* 2003). A frame helps us to make sense of complex information. It helps us interpret the world around us and represent that world to others. Frames help us organise complex phenomena into coherent, understandable categories. When we label a 'phenomenon' (a thing, an experience, a process) or something complex such as reflective practice, we give meaning to some aspects of what is observed, known or experienced, while discounting other aspects because they appear irrelevant or counter-intuitive. Thus, frames provide meaning through selective simplification. They also give us a field of vision for a problem.

For example, we might frame a thing such as a 'fast car' as one that goes from 0 to 60 mph in six seconds. An alternative 'framing' of this might be as a car that outperforms family saloon cars. Another framing might be concerned more with what a driver does with the car in particular road conditions. We might frame an experience such as a 'great party' as one where we were able to drink everything and anything we wanted, for free. Alternatively, it might be concerned more with meeting old friends or staying up late. Additionally, we might frame a process such as 'having a baby' in many ways – for example, in terms of the safe delivery of a healthy baby, in terms of being treated with kindness, respect and dignity, or in terms of having useful information so that we can make informed choices about where and how an individual has the baby.

Frames are built on values

Because frames are built upon our underlying values, intentions and experiences, we often find that frames about the same thing differ in significant ways. The process of framing involves both the construction of the frame and its representation or communication to others. In other words, we build personal interpretations of things, experiences and processes, and we advocate, teach or engage others with that preferred interpretation. Thatchenkery & Metzker (2006) put it this way:

> Framing is the psychological process whereby a person intentionally views or puts into a certain perspective any object, person, context or scenario. One of the most common examples of reframing is that of calling a glass half empty or half full. Regardless of how the glass is described, the amount of water is the same; it is only the perspective that is different.

(Thatchenkery & Metzker 2006, p. 6)

The perspective we may choose may depend upon whether you are 'an optimist or pessimist, dying of thirst or attempting to bail out a boat that is about to sink' (Thatchenkery & Metzker 2006, p. 6).

So, many factors influence our frames and their formation and communication to others. This also applies to the way we frame reflective practice, incorporate a particular frame within our various professional development programmes and communicate it to our staff, students or others at conferences. Three of the most common influences on the way we frame and re-frame things are our *identity*, the way we *characterise others* and issues of *power*. By re-framing, I mean shifts in both the frame itself and in its impact on others.

- *Our identity:* Every healthcare professional has a view of themselves. An identity in a specific clinical area or workplace. These identities spring from the individual's self-perception and team affiliation. If a particular framing of reflective practice (e.g. as public self-disclosure, of thoughts and feelings, with team colleagues) challenges one's sense of self, then the more oppositional we are likely to be to that particular frame. We may find it threatening to our sense of identity. This partially explains why the phrase 'reflective practice' has been greeted with a groan, an 'Oh, no!' or a sense of dread by students and colleagues. If a particular framing threatens us, then what happens? It can turn us away, reinforcing affiliations with like-minded individuals who share our framing of reflective practice (e.g. as a private activity, or as a set of tools, or as a whole disposition towards practice). We may also find that we negatively characterise those who hold alternative frames.
- *Characterising others:* Those who frame reflective practice in particular ways are often characterised (or stereotyped) by others. This characterisation may be either positive or negative: positive if the particular framing of reflective practice is aligned closely with your own values, purposes and intentions, and negative if not. Sometimes negative characterisations undermine the other's legitimacy. Sometimes this is done consciously and wilfully. Negative characterisations can cast doubt on others' motivations or be used to exploit their sensitivity. For example, if you believe in, and work with, a frame called 'self-reflection' and a mode of communicating this to others through story-telling or

narrative, you may be characterised (very negatively by some) as engaging in some kind of self-indulgent navel gazing. If your framing of reflective practice incorporates a sense of nurturing, intentional being and spirituality, then you may (by some) be characterised as engaging in some kind of 'touchy-feely' activity. If your framing of reflective practice is 'criticalist', then you may be regarded as a trouble-maker, a disruptive influence and someone to be avoided; if more emancipatory, then as utopian or structurally blind. An important root of such negative characterisations is knowing. If we think we already know what reflective practice is, the truth on the matter, then why do we need to listen to other people's views (or framing) of it? Talking openly about, and respectfully acknowledging, different ways to frame and practise reflection is what is needed. Talking in this way means being willing to expose *to* others what is inside us. If you accept this, then listening openly means being willing to expose ourselves to something new *from* others.

- *Power:* Arguably, different ways of framing reflective practice are associated with different conceptions of power, social influence and control. A framing of reflective practice that celebrates the power of human 'agency' is different from one that is more overtly 'political' and that foregrounds the influence of 'structure'. Agency refers to the capacity of you and me (social actors) to make a difference in the world. Structure refers to the enduring rules, patterns and institutions that provide the social context within which our actions take place. This is a topic of much debate. Briefly, this is why. Agency allows us to influence our social context, for example our healthcare work-places. So, the structures embodied in the organisation for which we work are an effect of agency (i.e. our actions). However, the argument runs the other way too. Because social, political, cultural, economic and other structures limit and constrain (some would argue deter-mine) our actions, agency (i.e. our actions) is also an effect of structure (i.e. the way our healthcare organisation works). Common sense sug-gests that both are partially true. The interplay between the power of human agency vis-à-vis the power of structure is the central topic of the agency-structure debate in social theory. It is a debate because of the dual purpose the theory can serve. That is, it can unseat the idea of structure as a dominant external influence on our actions and it can be used to deny the random character of human action. It can be used to argue that we are not merely puppets dancing to someone else's tune, and nor are we agents who are self-transparently aware of what we are doing. The power dimension, within our particular fram-ing of reflective practice, can advance or limit our own position and goals. It influences others' perceptions of our authority, our ability to secure resources (e.g. time and money) for reflective practice, our abil-ity to build coalitions, how threatening colleagues feel we might be, the way our voice gets heard in the boardroom, and so on.

Re-framing and scaling up reflection

So let's get back to the main issue, namely the suggestion that we need to consider re-framing reflection if we are to scale it up in the way I described earlier. At the scale of the individual reflective practitioner, Dewey (1933) framed reflection as a personal *disposition*. More recently this individualistic framing has focused on *mindfulness* (Johns 2004). Mindfulness is the development of our ability to pay deliberate attention to our experience, from moment to moment. It is attending to what is going on in our mind, body and day-to-day life, without judgement. It involves becoming more aware of our thoughts and feelings, but crucially suspending judgement and self-criticism. And the purpose? Many people have reported that it helps them find inner strengths and resources to enable them to make wise decisions about their health and life in general.

Reflective mindset

If we scale this up to workgroups and healthcare teams, I suggest we use the term 'reflective mindset'. This is an articulated set of values, relationships or ways of working that gives team members a strong sense of team identity and cohesion. A team's mindset creates a powerful incentive and rationale for its members to continue to adopt or accept prior behaviours, choices or tools. A shared mindset helps many teams to work well together and, when the task demands, to think and act as one. Arguably, it is supportive of high performance. The term 'mindset' should not be confused with 'groupthink'. This is a mode of thought (a frame) where members conform to what they perceive to be the consensus of the group. Groupthink may cause those involved to make irrational decisions, which each member might, individually, consider to be unwise.

Reflective mindscape

When thinking about reflection at the scale of the whole organisation, I suggest we frame using the term 'mindscape'. I have borrowed this term from the systems philosopher Maruyama (1980) and his early work, but I use it slightly differently. Mindscape is a powerful metaphor that conjures up visions of organisational 'landscapes of the mind'. It is a collective frame that takes in the whole system. I use the term 'mindscape' as a way of framing reflection at the systemic level. It is a term that can help us focus on systems-wide reflective habits of mind and habits of work. Maruyama identified four dominant mindscapes (hierarchical, independent, systemic and generative). In organisations, we might realistically talk about the most pervasive and acceptable organisational mindscape, rather than kidding ourselves that a mindscape is like an organisational blanket, snuffing out other competing or complementary kinds of mindscape. The same argument holds when we get drawn in to describing a trust's culture, when really we should be thinking about cultures with

Table 0.1 Some different ways to frame reflection and its alignment with scale and actions.

Who: learning by the . . .	Scale: focus on the . . .	Frame: broadly framed as . . .	Action: triggered by reflective questions such as . . .
Reflective practitioner	Individual	Mindfulness	How can I improve my practice, here, with this patient/client?
Reflective team	Collegial	Mindset	How can we improve our services for these particular patients/clients?
Reflective organisation	Collective	Mindscape	How can the trust provide high-quality, cost-effective services to all our customers?

one or more being dominant over time and in different directorates. As with the notion of mindset, we must guard against mindscapes becoming so organisationally embedded that they become resistant to change and transformation. If this happens, then a team's mindset and an organisation's mindscape may become yet another form of oppression. Put simply, a reflective organisational mindscape refers to the reflective habits of thought and actions of its workforce. Table 0.1 summarises the essence of different ways to broadly frame reflection.

What is r-learning?

R-learning is an intentional activity. It is learning that has four basic intentions. These are described as learning to:

- develop appreciations;
- (re-)frame experience;
- build collective wisdom;
- achieve and move forward.

These are explained in more detail below (see pp. 15–17).

The collective *characteristics* of r-learning are as follows. It is learning that is:

- *Appreciative:* It is learning that begins from a reflection on what works well, on success and the reasons for this. It is, therefore, a strength-based rather than a deficit-based approach. It searches for and celebrates the positive, what is valuable and constructive.

- *Generative:* It is derived from supported and collegial forms of reflection on experience that give us the opportunity and courage to see freshly and with eyes wide open. This re-framing is different from always seeing and understanding bounded by what we already know.
- *Transcending:* It arises from asking questions that really matter – the 'big questions' that help us better understand who we are and why we think and act in the ways we do; the 'serious questions' that help us transcend fear, force and failure, oppressive, exclusive and exploitative work practices; the 'positive questions' that help build a collective wisdom of values, intentions and actions. It is learning that is elevating, affirming and energising.
- *Transformative:* It accrues from the way reflection informs and transforms action and vice versa. This reciprocity provides the basis for useful learning. By this, I mean learning that can be put to good use in order to improve ourselves and the services we provide, for clients/patients, in particular settings. It helps us achieve something more or different. It is learning that helps us move forward.

Figure 0.2 is an attempt to bring these four basic intentions into a new wholeness called r-learning.

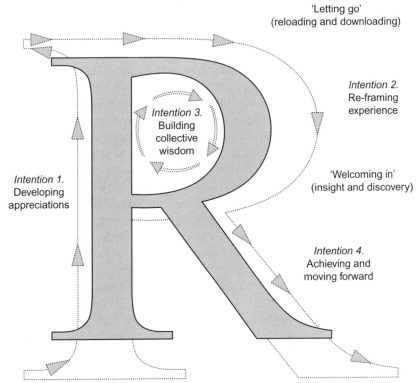

Figure 0.2   R-learning brought into wholeness.

The wholeness of r-learning

Figure 0.2 suggests that r-learning begins with *appreciation*; that is, learning that values the best of what is, of learning about individual and collective accomplishments. These appreciations begin virtuous upward learning spirals (rather than vicious downward spirals), which provide us with the confidence and courage to begin to learn more and different things by (re-)framing our developing experience. When learning in this way, we need a positive 'frame of mind' that focuses our energies on *welcoming in*, not on *closing out*. To do this we have to try to *let go* of two bad habits that distort the re-framing process. Kahane (2004) calls these habits *reloading* and *downloading*. Reloading is when we are not truly and openly attending to what's happening, not really listening, empathising or wanting to understand. What we are actually doing, when reloading, is rewinding some already existing mental tapes and rehearsing them in our mind. These are tapes that contain those things that we already know and ways we always behave. Downloading is when we reproduce (communicate) without alteration. There is no creativity associated with this. Downloading is no good for creating new insight and breakthroughs. When we download, we are deaf to others' stories and insensitive to other possibilities. We hear only that which confirms our own story. We listen, act and think from within our own, already existing experience. By *welcoming in*, I mean adopting a frame of mind that enables us to develop our *positive core* of values, intentions and actions that help us sustain and create new social realities. Unlike downloading (saying what we always say, doing what we always do, thinking in the same old ways), welcoming in is about listening to, and learning from, others who have a stake in the healthcare system. It is learning from those who have different, even opposing, perspectives to our own. These may be from those both inside and outside of healthcare. Welcoming in is about confronting the fact that we do not always know everything or the 'truth' about everything, confronting the fact that all knowledge has a sell-by date and that much of it is 'contested' (Phillips 2000). Welcoming in is wanting to develop new *insight* and experiencing the thrill of this. Fundamentally, it is learning that accrues from *discovering* what is new beyond your comfort zone. *Welcoming in* new insight, sensitivities, knowledge and skills enables us to (re-)frame experience and develop our positive core. This is indeed an *achievement*. In certain workplace contexts (cultures), we might be able to 'infect' others with these achievements; that is, to collectively improve how we are and what we can do, with and for others.

R-learning, then, is quite different from the kind of learning that is often pervasive in some healthcare organisations and clinical contexts where there is a constant state of stress, burden, anxiety and uncertainty, in workplaces where we constantly feel on the receiving end of yet more reforms, reforms that we had no hand in creating. In these workplaces, another kind of learning takes place. This is called *reactive learning*.

> Reactive learning is governed by 'downloading' habitual ways of thinking, of continuing to see the world from within the familiar categories we're comfortable with. We discard interpretations and options for action that are different from those we know and trust. We act to defend our interests. In reactive learning, our actions are actually re-enacted habits . . . Regardless of the outcome, we end up being 'right'. At best, we get better at what we have always done.

(Senge *et al.* 2005, pp. 10–11)

This is the antithesis of r-learning.

The book's basic action steps

The book is an attempt to think through ways of trying to build a reflective healthcare organisation. Taking this seriously suggests that the following five needs have to be satisfied:

- *Clarity:* We need to be clear about which intentions of reflection might be most supportive of building a reflective healthcare organisation. This clarity motivates us to act in a particular way.
- *Process:* We need a supportive, flexible and participatory force for change that is both aspirational and survivable given the complexity and pace of healthcare reform. We need a force that enables individual reflective practitioners to aggregate, to become communities of reflective practitioners within their own organisations.
- *Courage:* We need the courage to commit to action, put our values into practice, weigh up the risks and endure the hardships, and to do this ethically.
- *Knowledge:* We need to know how to generate, share and apply useful knowledge and different kinds of knowledge from within and outside of healthcare. In management-speak, this is called learning to 'wire for action'.
- *Learning:* We need to learn from our personal experiences and from each other and record these in some useful way so we can remind ourselves of where we have come from. Reflective learning starts with a conversation and needs to mature into genuine dialogue, where work teams and groups achieve more and different things compared with that attainable by the individual. We need to learn where and how to take action that leads to significant and enduring improvements.

So let us pull this together and get back to the central question of how to scale up reflective learning so that it becomes an organisation-wide frame of mind and work habit. In order to address this question, the book is organised into four fundamental action steps. Appreciating one step provides us with the reasons, capability and courage to take the next step. The action steps are:

Action step 1   Developing an appreciation of reflective learning
As mentioned earlier, reflection is a subject of much debate. In this first step I take some time to set out some of its more common conceptions and practices. I try to see these freshly. I start from some familiar, well-trodden ground and conclude with a broad re-framing of the field.

Action step 2   R-learning as an innovation
Understanding how we can scale up r-learning requires a deep appreciation of the notion of an innovation and the process of adoption.

Action step 3   Journeying along action pathways-to-scale
Here I describe six *action pathways* that enable us to progress towards a reflective organisation. These pathways are called values, conversation, user, leadership, team and network.

Action step 4   A force for change
With this final step, I put forward the case that RAISE is one particular force for change that is supportive of r-learning. RAISE contains five forces.

What is an action pathway?

I have taken the notion of an action pathway from the work of Redwood *et al.* (1999). In their work on action management, they argue that the key to successful action is to follow the right path. From a global action survey that they conducted, they identified four action paths and described the *action management* issues associated with each one. Each path differed in complexity and duration. They rather appealingly related their paths to different kinds of athletic event. Their action paths are:

- *The sprint:* a low-complexity, short-duration action path.
- *The high jump:* a high-complexity action of short duration.
- *The decathlon:* high-complexity actions of long duration.
- *The marathon:* a low-complexity action of long duration.

Essentially, they are saying that in order to move an organisation forward, it is wise to consider the factors that influence the *complexity* of one's action and then to consider those things that are likely to influence the *duration* of that action. The more people affected, the more complex the action is likely to be. The greater the performance improvement you seek, the more complex the action. When we turn our attention to duration, we soon appreciate that this is a very slippery idea. Duration is the amount of time the action is likely to take to achieve its goal. If the health-care organisation's mindscape is dominated by thoughts that there is never enough time and where 'early wins' are the name of the game, then

this becomes a thorny issue. In general, duration is likely to be determined by at least six interrelated, internal organisational characteristics:

- the nature of feedback and pressure from users of healthcare services;
- how quickly, safely and efficiently healthcare staff learn new ways of
  working;
- how understandable, and therefore compelling, your case is for new
  or preferred action;
- how long it took your organisation to complete something similar in
  the past;
- the current resources available;
- your present 'starting position' in relation to your desired goal.

For some, this is all about the amount of organisational culture change
involved.

Pathways-to-scale

In this book I set out six possible action pathways that enable us to make
progress towards building a reflective healthcare organisation. They
might be usefully regarded as *pathways-to-scale*. There is no right or
wrong pathway. Neither is there a predetermined sequence of pathways
to be followed. There is only what is right for your organisation, given
your assessment of its 'starting position'. Table 0.2 summarises the six
pathways.

More than one action pathway might have to be used in order to scale
up reflection from individual to organisation-wide practice. Some individual action pathways naturally link with and need others. In reality,
progress on one pathway becomes related to progress on another. By
reflecting on our action, I hope we will make wise choices about which
pathways are naturally and mutually supportive of each other. Which

Table 0.2 Six action pathways that enable us to make progress towards
building a reflective healthcare organisation.

Action pathway name	Reflection with action as . . .
Values	Developing an understanding and congruence between espoused and values-in-action
Conversation	Using the power of the positive question
User	Learning from patient and client experiences
Leadership	Leaders using their appreciative intelligence
Team	Learning shared within and between teams
Network	Linked groups working in a knowledge-sharing way

ones need and can sustain others? Which are best taken now and which later? Another genuine question emerges:

> What is or are your most appropriate path(s) that enable you to scale up reflective learning?

My suggestion is that the 'values pathway' is a very good place to start your journey.

Is it enough to know an action's path?

If we don't know where we are going, then any path will do. This is a truism. It's important that we don't take our eye off the vision, namely building a reflective organisation. It's also important that you know how far staff in your organisation will 'buy in' and support this vision. This depends on your ability to develop a credible case for it. In Table 0.3, I set out some further considerations that enable us to deepen our understanding of issues related to the complexity and duration of each action pathway-to-scale. In action step 3 of this book, I take each action pathway, elucidate its meaning and relate it to making progress towards building a reflective healthcare organisation.

Scaling up reflective learning: some challenges in taking action

In general this is a book about positive action, action that has a clear intention to improve something. It is committed action from individuals and workgroups, or teams, that supports the building of a reflective healthcare organisation. This is quite a challenge.

In 1996 PricewaterhouseCoopers conducted a survey of over 500 multinational businesses in 14 countries around the world. This involved high-technology and financial services, oil and healthcare. They undertook a global action survey that asked managers an important question: 'What barriers do you encounter when you take action and how do you overcome them?' They came up with ten major challenges (Redwood *et al*. 1999). See Table 0.4.

So, how can we scale up reflective learning so that it becomes a collegial and useful, organisation-wide, sustainable work habit?

You are right if you feel the book's central question has a rather futuristic tone. I admit the book is aspirational and hopeful. But it also tries to be realistic and practical. In order to work towards achieving this aspiration, I offer you a practical force for change. This force is called RAISE, which is grounded in practice and developed from IRP-UK's work undertaken both inside healthcare and beyond. The principle intention of RAISE is to enable organisations to scale up reflective learning. It requires those who commit to it to weave together *positive thinking* with *positive action*.

Table 0.3 Some attributes that determine the complexity and duration of each r-learning action pathway-to-scale.

Action pathway	Scaling up via this pathway requires a critical mass of . . .	Value position	Potential obstacles on the action pathway are . . .	Progress along action pathway sustained by . . .
Values	Staff with emotional intelligence	It is important to understand the moral purposes and the 'why' of change	Inability to articulate individual and collective values, tokenism and confusion	Congruence between espoused values and values-in-action
Conversation	Staff developing the organisation's 'positive core' through the use of the 'positive question'	Plan for an improved future based on what is right rather than what is wrong	Lack of trust, respect for others, promise-keeping and unfairness	Focusing on the root causes of success
User	Service users working to create improvements that matter to them	Healthcare services can be improved by actively listening and responding to service users	Users denied choice and control due to poor information and support	People throughout the system wanting to do their very best for service users
Leadership	Those with appreciative intelligence	Everything you do can make a positive difference	Action overload, depression, anger and inability to endure hardship	Leaders with persistence, conviction, tolerance for uncertainty, irrepressible resilience

(Continued)

Table 0.3 (Continued)

Action pathway	Scaling up via this pathway requires a critical mass of . . .	Value position	Potential obstacles on the action pathway are . . .	Progress along action pathway sustained by . . .
Team	Reflective teams sustained by supportive peer relationships and knowledge sharing	Working and learning together increases the likelihood that meaningful and useful change will occur	Perceptions of exclusivity, elitism and privilege	Quality and utility of reflective conversations
Network	Staff who can 'join up the dots', relate the parts to the bigger picture and develop understanding through coherence	Encourage more integrated ways of working and networked organisations	Poor communication systems, turf protection, cultures of disappointment and cynicism	Using the potential of appreciative knowledge sharing

Table 0.4   Ten challenges in taking action.

Challenge 1: plan for action	All action needs to be guided by a plan
Challenge 2: allocate for action	Effective action needs to be resourced appropriately
Challenge 3: lead for action	Action leading to improvement needs to be led well because much depends upon the exercise of power, influence and persuasion
Challenge 4: strengthen for action	Who or what needs to be strengthened if action leading to improvement is to stand a chance?
Challenge 5: mobilise for action	Action needs enthusiasm and motivated people to initiate and keep it going
Challenge 6: clarify for action	If you haven't explained to staff why they need to act differently, they are unlikely to change what they are currently doing
Challenge 7: cultivate for action	Better, rather than simply different, action requires an understanding of each person's gifts and talents
Challenge 8: integrate for action	Action for improvement often requires new and different ways of working to overcome functional barriers ('We do this, in this way, here') and cultural barriers ('This is why we do what we do, every day, with those with whom we work and for whom we care')
Challenge 9: wire for action	Some action requires the support of modern (information) technologies. Fast, accurate, useable, well-managed information (knowledge) systems are required
Challenge 10: re-energise for action	Any action takes energy. Energy management and renewal are important to combat fatigue

(Redwood *et al.* 1999)

Thus far, we have a vision – that of building a reflective healthcare organisation. We know that such an organisation is supported and sustained by four r-learning intentions. We also have six action pathways (or routes) that help us make progress towards achieving this vision. What we need now is a force for change, something that will enable us to scale up r-learning from an individual pursuit to an organisation-wide work habit. We need a positive force that helps us acknowledge where we've come from (looking over our shoulder), appreciate current achievements (acknowledging the positive present) and embrace the challenges of the next steps (looking forward).

RAISE is one such positive force for change. Participants using RAISE need a commitment to make it work. This is fundamentally about trust. If staff lack trust in things, in each other and in change processes, then they can become suspicious, hostile, half-hearted, anxious or uncertain. When individuals and groups feel this way, it is unlikely that they will allow themselves, emotionally, cognitively or practically, to be caught up in RAISE or any other change process. What is required to achieve this vision is at least:

- a positive 'can do' or 'will try to' attitude rather than a (jaded or tired) 'can't do' or 'it won't work here' attitude;
- a general acceptance that organisational health and wellbeing at work depend on how people feel just as much as what they do;
- a journey that is survivable even though it may require those involved to change aspects of how they currently feel, think and act. The individual and collective self-awareness required for this to happen is crucial to making positive progress along a chosen action pathway.

RAISE

RAISE is a force for change with two meanings. First, it is a word in its own right and with a clear action orientation. It is meant to convey a sense of 'raising the bar', of elevating learning through reflection by moving it from the individual to the systemic. RAISE is about promoting and actively enhancing this. No simple task! RAISE also alludes to raising the collective reflective pulse (raising a head of steam), raising the voices of all stakeholders, often raising people's courage and spirits for such action. But all this for what? Well, we now know reflective learning can bring with it:

- deeper appreciations;
- increased individual and collective re-framing capabilities;
- more courage and clarity of thinking to confront and improve con-structed workplace realities and develop our positive core of values and practices and build collective wisdom;
- an improvement orientation that provides us with the courage and capacity to move forward.

(See pp. 14–17 for an elaboration of these four claims.)

Second, RAISE is an acronym. It is words within a word. Its parts describe the particular forces that need to operate in order to scale up r-learning:

R = *reflecting*
The need to reflect on our experiences and learn from our practice. The emphasis needs to be on the creation of a positive core of values and

actions and, additionally, on the creation of 'texts' (reflective accounts of one kind or another) that help us to better understand ourselves, our work and workplace and enable us to make wise decisions about how to move forward. Texts help us develop a sense of history. They chart our progress. Done well, texts leave positive footprints that enable us to understand how we have come to be where we are today.

A = appreciating

The need to develop cultures of appreciation where current strengths and achievements (the 'positive present') form the basis for an improved future. Appreciative organisational healthcare cultures focus consciously on success rather than only on 'fixing' those things that are going wrong.

I = interacting

Scaling up quality interactions (patterns of behaviour and kinds of conversation) to the collective level (workgroup, team, department, unit, clinic, hospital, community, etc.) that are strength-based and creative. This is about scaling up conversations that are improvement-oriented and positively embrace the dynamic, generative and social complexities of the 'rough ground' of practice and policy development.

S = strategising

In order to be successful, scaling up r-learning cannot be a hit-and-miss affair. It needs to be a planned process. Another way of putting this is that it requires a strategy. Strategising is the process of strategy formation. Many forces influence this process. An important one is the use of power.

E = energising

Any scaling up of reflective learning (any action) takes energy. Full engagement necessitates careful energy management and renewal. This is important in order to combat action overload and fatigue. Individual and collective 'recovery plans' are crucial. The larger and more complex the scaling up process, the longer it takes and the greater the possibility that boredom or fatigue will get in the way. Fatigue shows itself in many ways, for example in people's inability to focus on the organisation's vision and to keep their eye on its underlying purpose, apparent disinterest, and an inability to take the scaling-up process seriously.

Mapping out the 'rough ground'

The two main metaphors used in this book are those of 'rough ground' and a 'journey'.

A metaphor helps us make sense of something complex or unfamiliar (Chapman 2002, Hunt 2001, 2006, Perry & Cooper 2001, Ritchie & Rigano 2007). Metaphors are very useful. A metaphor gives a name to something that belongs to something else. For example, learning how to drive a car in an urban area is like a game of chess. 'Chess' is used as the metaphor. Chess 'pieces' are cars of different sizes and shapes that do different things. The rules of the chess game link with the rules of the Highway

Code that determine what you can and can't do. Chess is a game of unexpected moves and surprises that have to be 'countered' by the other player. On the road, good drivers have to react safely to the unexpected, the surprises and the dangers.

How far could the metaphor of 'crossroads' help you reflect upon some of the most important decisions you have had to make in your personal or professional life, decisions that have given your life the direction it has thus far? How far does the metaphor of 'mountain climbing' help you reflect on and describe your professional life? How far do the metaphors of 'juggling' or 'nurturing' help you reflect upon the work that you do?

In his book *Educating the Reflective Practitioner*, Schön (1987) uses the metaphor of the swamp and the high ground:

> On the high ground, manageable problems lend themselves to solution through the application of research-based theory and technique. In the swampy lowland, messy, confusing problems defy technical solution.

(Schön 1987, p. 3)

Without doubt, life in the swamp, with the 'messy and confusing problems' of practice, can lead to powerful opportunities for learning. If we take on the arguments mentioned earlier about the power of human agency, then we can say that here we have at least two choices: to climb out of the swamp and stay on the high ground, or to descend from the high ground into the swamp and maybe stay there. In embracing the challenges of building the reflective healthcare organisation, another metaphor may be more useful.

The rough ground of reflective practice

It is Wittgenstein's metaphor of 'rough ground' (Blair 2006), captured in a 1993 Derek Jarman film of the Viennese-born, Cambridge-educated philosopher Ludwig Wittgenstein (1889–1951), that I have in mind. In essence, this metaphor is all about 'friction'. When we try to walk on slippery ice, where there is no friction, we are unable to do so. We fall over. If we want to walk, we need an amount of friction. In Jarman's film, Wittgenstein's image of the 'crystalline purity of logic' is set in contrast with the 'rough ground' of what we actually say and do. As the film unfolds, a young man dreams of reducing the world to pure logic. It's a dream of a world purged of imperfection and Schön-like indeterminacy. The world becomes a landscape of gleaming ice. But this world, perfect though it might seem, is uninhabitable because it is a landscape without friction. When he is older, the man begins to appreciate that roughness, ambiguity, error and indeterminacy are not simply deficits and imperfections; they are an important part of life and what actually makes things work. He begins to dig up the ice to uncover the rough ground, but he can't sustain this. He yearns for the ice, where everything appears radiant and absolute. Unable to live on the rough ground, he ends up marooned between earth and ice, at home in neither. As we move into action step 1 of this book, we begin to (re-)discover some of this 'rough ground of reflective practice'.

References

Blair, D. (2006) *Wittgenstein, Language and Information: 'Back to the Rough Ground!'*. Springer-Verlag, New York.

Buzan, T. (2006) *The Ultimate Book of Mind Maps*. HarperThorsons, London.

Chapman, V. (2002) Teaching as a site of re-presentation: metaphors, tropes and texts. *Reflective Practice* **3**(2), 191–204.

Department of Health (2006) Good doctors, safer patients: proposals to strengthen the system to assure and improve the performance of doctors and to protect the safety of patients. A report by the Chief Medical Officer, July 2006. Department of Health, London. Available at www.dh.gov.uk/PublicationsAndStatistics/Publications/PublicationsPolicyAndGuidance/PublicationsPolicyAndGuidanceArticle/fs/en? CONTENT_ID=4137232&chk=KW63va

Dewey, J. (1933) *How We Think: A Restatement of the Relation of Reflective Thinking to the Educative Process*. Heath and Company, Lexington, MA.

Fullan, M. (2004) Systems thinkers in action: moving beyond the standards plateau. Available at http://publications.teachernet.gov.uk/eOrderingDownload/Systems%20Thinkers%20in%20Action.pdf.

Goldratt, E.M. (1990) *What is this Thing Called Theory of Constraints and How Should it be Implemented?* North River Press, Corton-on-Hudson, NY.

Gonos, G. (1997) 'Situation' versus 'frame': the 'interactionist' and the 'structuralist' analyses of everyday life. *American Sociological Review* **42**, 854–67.

Gray, B. (1989) *Collaborating: Finding Common Ground for Multiparty Problems*. Jossey-Bass, San Francisco, CA.

Hunt, C. (2001) Shifting shadows: metaphors and maps for facilitating reflective practice. *Reflective Practice* **2**(3), 275–87.

Hunt, C. (2006) Travels with a turtle: metaphors and the making of a professional identity. *Reflective Practice* **7**(3), 315–32.

Johns, C. (2002) *Guided Reflection: Advancing Practice*. Blackwell Science, Oxford.

Johns, C. (2004) *Being Mindful, Easy Suffering: Reflections on Palliative Care*. Jessica Kingsley Publishers, London.

Kahane, A. (2004) *Solving Tough Problems: An Open Way of Talking, Listening and Creating New Realities*. Berrett-Koehler, San Francisco, CA.

Kahneman, D. & Tversky, A. (1979) Prospect theory: an analysis of decision under risk. *Econometrica* **47**, 263–89.

Lewicki, R., Gray, B. & Elliott, M. (2003) *Making Sense of Intractable Environmental Conflicts: Concepts and Cases*. Island Press, Washington, DC.

Maruyama, M. (1980) Mindscapes and science theories. *Current Anthropology* **21**, 589–99.

Minsky, M. (1975) A framework for representing knowledge. In *The Psychology of Computer Vision* (ed. P.H. Winston). McGraw-Hill, New York.

Neale, M.A. & Bazerman, M.H. (1985) The effects of framing and negotiator overconfidence on bargaining behaviours and outcomes. *Academy of Management Journal* **28**, 34–49.

Nursing and Midwifery Council (2006) Clinical supervision: A–Z advice sheet. Available at www.nmc-uk.org/aFrameDisplay.aspx?DocumentID=1558

Paton, N. (2006) Divided loyalties. *Nursing Times* **102**(24), 18–19.

Perry, C. & Cooper, M. (2001) Metaphors are good mirrors: reflecting on change for teacher education. *Reflective Practice* **7**(1), 41–52.

Phillips, J. (2000) *Contested Knowledge: A Guide to Critical Theory*, 2nd edn. Zed Books, London.

Pinkley, R.L. (1990) Dimensions of conflict frame: disputant interpretations of conflict. *Journal of Applied Psychology* **75**, 117–26.

Redwood, S., Goldwasser, C., Street, S. & PricewaterhouseCoopers LLP (1999) *Action Management*. John Wiley & Sons, New York.

Ritchie, S. & Rigano, D. (2007) Writing together metaphorically and bodily side-by-side: an inquiry into collaborative academic writing. *Reflective Practice* **8**(1), 123–35.

Schön, D. (1987) *Educating the Reflective Practitioner: Towards a New Design for Teaching and Learning in the Professions*. Jossey-Bass, San Francisco, CA.

Seligman, M.E.P. (2006) *Learned Optimism: How to Change Your Mind and Your Life*. Vintage Books, New York.

Senge, P. (1990) *The Fifth Discipline: The Art and Practice of Organizational Learning*. Doubleday, New York.

Senge, P., Scharmer, C., Jaworski, J. & Flowers, B. (2005) *Presence: An Exploration of Profound Change in People, Organizations and Society*. Doubleday, New York.

Taylor D.E. (2000) The rise of the environmental justice paradigm: injustice framing and the social construction of environmental discourses. *American Behavioral Scientist* **43**(4), 508–80.

Thatchenkery, T. & Metzker, C. (2006) *Appreciative Intelligence: Seeing the Mighty Oak in the Acorn*. Berrett-Koehler, San Francisco, CA.

Van de Ven, A.H., Polley, D., Garud, R. & Venkataraman. S. (1999) *The Innovation Journey*. Oxford University Press, New York and Oxford.

van Manen, M. (1999) The practice of practice. In *Changing Schools, Changing Practices: Perspectives on Educational Reform and Teacher Professionalism* (ed. M. Lang). Garant, Luvain, Belgium.

Watzlawick, P., Weakland, J. & Fisch, R. (1974) *Change, Principles of Problem Formation and Problem Resolution*. Norton, New York.

Young, A. (2006) Finding time to reflect. *Nursing Times* **102**(32), 22.

Chapter 1

Action step 1: developing an appreciation of reflective learning

In this first step on to the 'rough ground', I begin by walking in some of the footsteps of others. I do this because I wish to establish in your mind a positive appreciation of the way reflective practice has, until now, been more widely conceived and used. Later I re-frame and extend these conceptions by drawing attention to the ways reflective learning (rather than practice) as a collective and political process (not method) can support service and organisational development.

Action step 1 contains six major *ideas bundles*:

Bundle 1   **Conceptions**
This invites you to think about the image(s) that the words 'reflection' and 'reflective practice' conjure up in your mind. It also includes the idea that there are many kinds of reflection.

Bundle 2   **Practices of reflection**
There are not only many kinds of reflection but also many ways to practise it. This bundle sets out reflection as a conscious, intentional, creative and critical work habit.

Bundle 3   **Frameworks for action**
This includes four kinds of framework (or 'model') for supporting and guiding reflection. They are frameworks comprising questions, stages, levels and cycles.

Bundle 4   **The reflective practitioner**
This embraces the essence of the work of some principal writers on the subject, such as Schön, Dewey, Mezirow, Zeichner & Liston, Day and Pollard. It develops our appreciation of the (historical) pervasiveness of reflection as an individualistic practice.

Bundle 5   **Getting organised**
This involves stepping on to relatively new ground by thinking about some influences on getting organised for scaling up reflection. The important influences of workplace cultures and the quality of workplace learning are included in this bundle.

Bundle 6   **Re-framing reflective practices**
Action step 1 concludes with an attempt to re-frame earlier appreciations of the nature of reflection and the practices of it. An analysis of the content, processes and shifting foci, contained in 512 academic papers, provides an opportunity to link four principle intentions of the practices of reflection with their use at different scales. Collectively, we can think of this as a meta-analysis.

To help you navigate your way through action step 1, these ideas bundles are linked together into a mind map (Fig. 1.1).

Some conceptions of reflective practice

The nature of reflection and reflective practice is a subject of much debate. There are a range of conceptions, a variety of practices and 'internal disputes'. I am concerned that as reflective practice continues to be 'fashionable', four things are happening. The first is that any kind of 'practice' that involves 'thinking again about my work' gets labelled as reflective practice. So, anything from snatched moments during a coffee break, to leisurely walks with the dog, where the mind wanders into thinking again about some aspect of what we might have done or observed at work, gets called reflective practice. Sometimes it is labelled with a term such as clinical supervision, mentoring or coaching. Often the label obscures the underlying process (reflection) and the positive core value (learning). Sometimes reflective practices get embedded within leadership programmes and lifelong learning and form a vital part of action learning sets. Just like clinical governance, reflective practice gets interwoven into the fabric of the organisation. Arguably, it is not the label but the process that is important. On an optimistic note, there may exist far more reflective healthcare organisations than we might imagine.

Second, the attention on reflective *practice* (singular) has the distorting effect of emphasising methods and techniques. It skews attention towards 'how to do it' rather than 'how to live by it'. Third, this distortion puts the potential to make a difference, which reflection brings with it, at risk because it loosens (or even uncouples) reflection from learning. Fourth, there is a danger that we may become 'fashion victims' (Ghaye & Lillyman 2000) if we develop an overzealous attention to reflective practice without any clear and considered justification of or for its use or any real understanding of its potential to enable us to:

- develop appreciations;
- (re-)frame experience;
- build a collective wisdom of values, intentions and actions;
- achieve and move forward.

These potentials should not be acknowledged uncritically.

The evidence-base for action step 1

Until now, there has been a developing appreciation in the helping and caring professions that the practices of reflection, if done systematically,

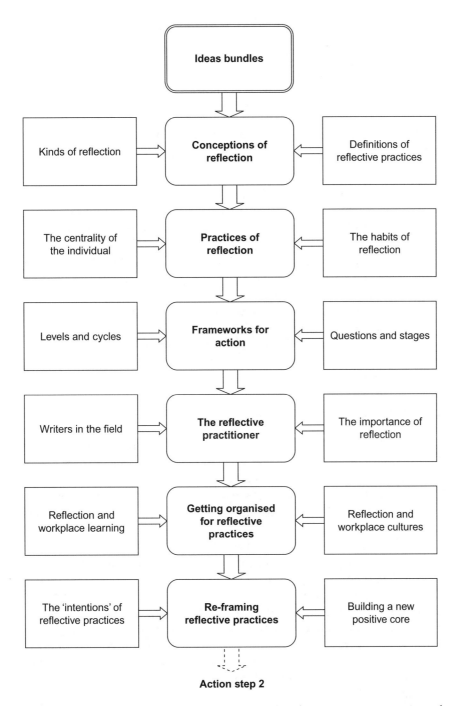

Figure 1.1 A mind map for action step 1: developing an appreciation of reflective learning.

rigorously, collectively and publicly, can and do lead to improvements in individual

- feelings about work and working life;
- thoughts about work and working life;
- actions in particular workplaces.

The evidence-base for such appreciations is derived from four main sources:

- 25 years of personal observation and interaction with individuals and teams across a spectrum of human service work;
- the published experiences of people working in real-world caring contexts and disseminated in book form, some recent examples of which are shown in Table 1.1;
- the rise in the number of national and international conferences and websites that have reflective practices as a significant part of their focus (see Tables 1.2 and 1.3);
- the large and compelling volume of evidence accumulated in the international peer-reviewed journal *Reflective Practice*. Since the launch of this journal in 2000, 562 papers have been submitted for review. The journal publishes four issues per year.

Some conceptions of reflection

You may like to think about some views you hold of reflection. One may be captured by the word 'mirror'. This might make reflective practices a process where you see yourself reflected back at you. So does this mean you are what you see? Can you sense any problems with this view, for example around issues such as our tendency to see only what we want to see?

Another view may be captured by the word 'waterfall'. For example, how far do your feelings of engaging in reflection bring back feelings of fear or danger, of turmoil or mental or emotional turbulence? Still water becomes stagnant over time. Practice can also become stagnant if we don't keep it moving forward, if we don't turn it over and 'oxygenate' it. Today in healthcare, developing our practice has to be a visible process. We have to demonstrate it clearly to others. It can't be hidden away from view. We also have to provide evidence that we are moving forward. This can be in many forms, such as in a portfolio (Ghaye & Lillyman 2006b).

Engaging in reflective practices may be a bit like moving through a professional landscape of hills and high ground, of lowlands and swampy ground. How far does this connect with any views you may have about reflective practice? Is the high hard ground *the* place to be, to work? What might (working) life be like in the swampy lowlands?

Table 1.1 Focus of some recent books on reflective practice.

Author	Date	Title	Publisher	ISBN
Jasper, M.	2007	*Vital Notes for Nurses: Professional Development, Reflection and Decision-Making*	Blackwell Publishing	1405132612
Bradley, A.	2006	*Personal Development and Reflective Practice in a Learning Disability Service*	Bild Publications	1904082971
Dolan, P. *et al.* (eds)	2006	*Family Support as Reflective Practice*	Jessica Kingsley Publishers	1843103206
Ghaye, T. & Lillyman, S.	2006	*Learning Journals and Critical Incidents: Reflective Practice for Health Care Professionals, 2nd edn*	Mark Allen Publishing	185642331X
Hay, J.	2006	*Reflective Practice and Supervision for Coaches*	Open University Press	0335220630
Johns, C.	2006	*Engaging Reflection in Practice*	Blackwell Publishing	1405149736
York-Barr, J. *et al.*	2006	*Reflective Practice to Improve Schools: An Action Guide for Educators*	Corwin Press	1412917573
Beirne, M.	2005	*Empowerment and Innovation: Managers, Principles and Reflective Practice*	Edward Elgar Publishing	1843762463
Bolton, G.	2005	*Reflective Practice: Writing and Professional Development*	Sage Publications	1412908124
Ghaye, T.	2005	*Developing the Reflective Healthcare Team*	Blackwell Publishing	1405105917
Johns, C. & Freshwater, D. (eds)	2005	*Transforming Nursing through Reflective Practice*	Blackwell Publishing	1405114576
Pollard, A.	2005	*Reflective Teaching: Evidence Informed Professional Practice, 2nd edn*	Continuum	0826473954
Sergiovanni, T.J.	2005	*The Principalship: A Reflective Practice Perspective*	Allyn and Bacon	0205457231

(Continued)

Table 1.1 (Continued)

Author	Date	Title	Publisher	ISBN
Taylor, B.	2005	*Reflective Practice: A Guide for Nurses and Midwives, 2nd rev. edn*	Open University Press	0335217427
Bulman, C.	2004	*Reflective Practice in Nursing: The Growth of the Professional Practitioner*	Blackwell Publishing	1405111127
Farrell, T.S.C.	2004	*Reflective Practice in Action: 80 Reflection Breaks for Busy Teachers*	Corwin Press	0761931643
Ghaye, A. & Ghaye, K.	2004	*Teaching and Learning through Critical Reflective Practice*	David Fulton Press	185346548 8
Johns, C.	2004	*Becoming a Reflective Practitioner*	Blackwell Publishing	1405118334
Osterman, K.F.	2004	*Reflective Practice for Educators: Professional Development to Improve Student Learning*	Corwin Press	0803968019
Jasper, M.	2003	*Foundations in Nursing and Healthcare: Beginning Reflective Practice*	Nelson Thornes	0748771174
Ghaye, T. & Lillyman, S.	2000	*Caring Moments: The Discourse of Reflective Practice*	Mark Allen Publishing	1856421260
Ghaye, T. & Lillyman, S.	2000	*Effective Clinical Supervision: The Role of Reflection*	Mark Allen Publishing	1856421252
Ghaye, T. & Lillyman, S.	2000	*Reflection: Principles and Practice for Healthcare Professionals*	Mark Allen Publishing	1856421112
Ghaye, T., Lillyman, S. & Gillespie, D. (eds)	2000	*Empowerment through Reflection: The Narratives of Healthcare Professionals*	Mark Allen Publishing	1856420434

Table 1.2 Some conferences that have focused on reflective practice.

Conference	Host	Date	Venue
ALISE Annual Conference: Habits of Mind and Practice – Preparing Reflective Professionals	Association for Library and Information Science Education (ALISE)	15–18 January 2007	Seattle, WA, USA
Extending Professionalism, Improving Practice: Exploring the Impact of Action Research	Collaborative Action Research Network (CARN)	10–12 November 2006	University of Nottingham, Nottingham, UK
Practice Development, Action Research and Reflective Practice, 6th International Conference: Enhancing Practice 6 – Innovation, Creativity, Patient Care and Professionalism	Collaborative Action Research Network (CARN), Foundation of Nursing Studies (UK), Royal College of Nursing (RCN) Institute Practice Development Function (UK), Developing Practice Network (UK), University of Ulster (UK), Monash University (Australia), James Cook University (Australia), Victoria University of Wellington (New Zealand), Fontys University (the Netherlands), Northern Sydney Central Coast Health (Australia), Waikato District Health Board (New Zealand)	18–20 October 2006	Edinburgh Conference Centre, Heriot-Watt University, Edinburgh, UK

(Continued)

Table 1.2 (Continued)

Conference	Host	Date	Venue
Clinical Supervision and Reflective Practice in Prison	Centre for Excellence in Applied Research Mental Health	11 September 2006	Prison Service College, Rugby, UK
Professional Lifelong Learning: Beyond Reflective Practice	Standing Conference on University Teaching and Research in the Education of Adults (SCUTREA)	3 July 2006	Trinity & All Saints College, Leeds, UK
12th International Conference: The Reflective Practice Conference – Being and Intention in Health and Educational Care	University of Westminster in collaboration with Professor Christopher Johns and University of Luton	3–5 July 2006	Robinson College, Cambridge, UK
Demonstrating Competence Through Reflective Writing	International Institute of Reflective Practice-UK	2 February 2006	National Motorcycle Museum, Birmingham, UK
Third Annual Enhancement Themes Working Conference: The Reflective Sector Supporting Reflective Practice	Enhancement Themes	27 January 2006	University of Dundee, Dundee, UK
11th Cambridge International Conference on Open and Distance Learning: Reflective Practice in Open and Distance Learning – How Do We Improve?	International Research Foundation for Open Learning (IRFOL)	20–23 September 2005	University of Cambridge, UK

Title	Organizer	Date	Location
Scenario-Based Learning: Reflection and Action on Lived and Unlived Experiences	International Institute of Reflective Practice-UK	23–24 June 2005	Gloucester, UK
Reflective Practice: The Key to Innovation in International Education	Centre for Research in International Education	23–26 June 2005	Asquith Avenue Campus of AIS St Helens, Auckland, New Zealand
5th Annual International Reflective Practice Research Group Conference: Unanticipated Learning Outcomes and Reflective Practice	International Reflective Practice Research Group	19–22 May 2005	La Sapienza University, Rome, Italy
5th Creativity and Cognition Conference: Creative Process and Artefact Creation – Practice, Digital Media and Support Tools	Goldsmiths College, London; Creative and Cognition Studios in cooperation with ACM SIGCHI	12–15 April 2005	Goldsmiths College, University of London, UK
Association for Learning Technology (ALT) Spring Conference and Research Seminar 2005: Reflective Learning, Future Thinking	ALT in association with Irish Learning Technology Association (ILTA) and SURF	31 March 2005	Dublin Institute of Technology, Dublin, Ireland

(Continued)

Table 1.2 (Continued)

Conference	Host	Date	Venue
3rd Carfax International Conference on Reflective Practice: Reflection as a Catalyst for Change	International Institute of Reflective Practice-UK in association with Carfax, Taylor & Francis	23–25 June 2004	Gloucester, UK
4th Annual International Reflective Practice Research Group Conference: Reflective Practices – Mechanisms for Learning	International Reflective Practice Research Group	15–17 April 2004	University College, Bergen, Norway
2nd Carfax International Conference on Reflective Practice: Investing in Success – Reflection-with-Action	International Institute of Reflective Practice-UK in association with Carfax, Taylor & Francis	5–8 July 2002	Gloucester, UK
1st Carfax International Conference on Reflective Practice: Making a Difference through Reflective Practice – Values and Action	University of Worcester in association with Carfax, Taylor & Francis	13–16 July 2000	University of Worcester, Worcester, UK

Table 1.3 Some websites that focus on reflective practice.

Website	Web address
Chartered Society of Physiotherapy: Continuing Professional Development: Reflective Practice	www.csp.org.uk/director/careersandlearning/continuingprofessionaldevelopment/reflectivepractice.cfm
Douglas College: Reflective Practice Toolkit	www.development.douglas.bc.ca/teaching/welcome.html
Flying Start NHS – Reflective Practice	www.flyingstart.scot.nhs.uk/ReflectivePractice.htm
Gillie Bolton	www.gilliebolton.com
Institute of Reflective Practice-UK	www.reflectivepractices.co.uk
International Reflective Practice Research Group	http://condiscipuli.org.uk/
Love Health – Reflective Practice	www.lovehealth.org/tools/reflection.htm
Practice-Based Learning	www.practicebasedlearning.org/resources/reflection/intro.htm
National Capital Language Resource Center (NCLRC), Washington: What Language Teaching is: Reflective Teaching Practice	www.nclrc.org/essentials/whatteach/reflect.htm
Queensland University of Technology, Australia – Reflect – Reflective Happiness	www.reflectivehappiness.com
Reflective Practice	https://olt.qut.edu.au/it/REFLECT/index.cfm?fa=displayPage&rNum=1639183
Reflective Practitioner: Professional Mastery through Model Building	www.reflectivepractitioner.com
Standards Site, Department for Education & Skills – Reflective Practice	www.standards.dfes.gov.uk/innovation-unit/Information/ourprojects1/denemagna1/?version=1
UK Centre for Legal Education (UKCLE): Developing Reflective Practice in Legal Education	www.ukcle.ac.uk/resources/reflection/index.html
University of Alabama: Area of Teacher Education – Elementary Education Program: Reflective Practice	www.bamaed.ua.edu/~kstaples/Reflectivity.htm

Does being on hard high ground bring with it a sense of safety, stability or advantage? A feeling of superiority, of looking downwards at the world from above? A feeling of distance and perspective? And what about trying to make sense of everything from the messiness (Ackoff 1979) of the swamp? How far can you lift up your head when in the swampy lowland and see where you are going? Maybe you can't because you are too concerned about your next step. What might it be like to work where you continuously feel 'bogged down', where you dare not look up for fear of what you might see (yet more bog to get through), where progress is painfully slow? But can you see advantages of being in the swamp? Of positively embracing messiness?

Slow down, not speed up

In today's rapidly developing health services, many managers feel that fast decisions and quick implementation are what counts. But many issues and situations are new to us. Issues concerned with a patient-led NHS, commissioning, choice, payment by results and re-validation are new. Meaningful ways to engage positively with excluded groups – not only children but also adults, mental health service users and people with learning disabilities – are new. Developing ways to enable children (under age 16 years) to become governors of children's trusts is new. In these situations, slowing down (wading carefully through the complexities and challenges in the swamp) is a necessity. This is not a comfortable message for healthcare reformers. Slow down. Reflect. Observe. Position yourself. Marshal your arguments and evidence. Then act fast and with the confidence that comes from such conscious and deliberate reflections. We have to slow down long enough to see what's really needed.

> With a freshness of vision, we have the possibility of a freshness of action, and the overall response on a collective level can be much quicker than trying to implement hasty decisions that aren't compelling to people.
>
> (Senge *et al.* 2005, p. 86)

Is this reflection as ethical practice?

What follows now is a view of reflection from a third-year nursing student. After reading it through, ask yourself what are some of the:

- positive aspects (if any);
- worrying aspects (if any)

of this description of reflection?

> As students we are expected to fill our portfolios with reflections on our nursing experiences. This includes writing about things that upset us, reflecting upon possible triggers and how we felt afterwards.

I remember leaning against the door of the sluice with my fingers in my ears to drown out the sound of an elderly patient calling again and again for her dead mother, who she swore had just gone to the corner shop.

I remember becoming nauseated when entering the room of a dying patient and being transported back to the age of 11 when I had experienced the same smell in my father's room at the hospice.

These incidents affected me but I dealt with them professionally. I showed empathy, sorrow and used appropriate body language.

My husband and best friend are the only two people I wish to confide in. My feelings are private – yet I am expected to frame them in prose and submit them to my university.

I don't know my lecturers or personal tutor intimately. What right has any-one to ask for such personal information, let alone ask that it be graded by a faceless lecturer?

As nurses we respect patient's rights not to disclose their personal feelings. Yet no such right is afforded to students. I have had reflections returned with requests for more details about my feelings. I comply but deeply resent being asked to do so.

(Sinclair-Penwarden 2006, p. 12)

Are definitions of reflective practices important?

There are many definitions available. Arguably they are helpful because they illustrate the breadth of ideas and processes that have been caught up by the term. One definition rarely captures everything. Here are four examples:

Reflection is an active, persistent and careful consideration of any belief or sup-posed form of knowledge in the light of the grounds that support it and the further conclusions to which it tends.

(Dewey 1933, p. 118)

. . . critical reflection . . . using the reflective process to look systematically and rigorously at our own practice. We all reflect on our practice to some extent, but how often do we employ those reflections to learn from our actions, to challenge established theory and, most importantly, to make a real difference to practice?

(Rolfe *et al.* 2001, p. xi)

Reflection, as a process, seems to lie somewhere around the notion of learning and thinking. We reflect in order to learn something, or we learn as a result of reflecting – so 'reflective learning' as a term simply emphasises the intention to learn as a result of reflection.

(Moon 2004, p. 80)

Guided reflection is a process of self-enquiry to enable the practitioner to realise desirable and effective practice within a reflexive spiral of being and becoming . . . Being in guided reflection groups is reminiscent of the 'campfire' approach to storytelling, reflecting on our own wisdom as practitioners, giving voice to our personal knowing, ideas and opinions, learning to dialogue, and working our stories into the caring-healing tradition of nursing and healthcare.

(Johns 2002, p. 3)

I would argue that you should not spend too much time hunting out the 'perfect' definition but seek to find out how reflection is used in practice. By analysing what people do, important workplace-based and profession-specific definitions will emerge. These might be more useful to you. What is clear from these four statements is that reflective practices can be viewed as a catalyst for learning and a response to learning. You can, of course, choose to reflect on and learn from successful events in your work, or from failures and problems. Success and failure are two extremes.

Reflections on the failure-to-success spectrum

Reflective practices are often used to 'work on' failings or problems. Sometimes we have to remind ourselves that reflective practices can be used to strengthen successes as well. Failure, fear of it and problems, can be powerful forces for changing what we do. We may be inclined to reflect more readily on past problems and failures. We may feel these are the things we need to prioritise and 'fix'. Our 'failings' may require urgent attention. This may be perfectly justified. Sometimes failures or problems stimulate a greater willingness or readiness to consider alternatives. Failures can encourage us to be more critical of the way we currently do things. Sometimes failures and problems are linked with personal issues such as denial, avoiding risk, self-protection and defensiveness. These are tricky things that often need sorting out. Failures and problems are only two sources of motivation for changing our practice, however. Another is to learn from our successes and those things you feel you do best. So what do you do really well? Like failures, successes should not be left unexamined. They need to be reflected upon. This is because our success might be limited to a particular task or activity, or to an individual or group. By reflecting on 'significant incidents', we can learn to notice and appreciate the successful aspects of our work, no matter how small. These often go unnoticed. If recorded, these successes can create positive memories for us. These can balance personal feelings of frustration, which we may experience, when trying to develop our competence.

We can position any significant event we care to reflect upon somewhere between the two extremes of success and failure. Often in our daily work 'being good enough' or 'doing the best we can' is all we can hope for. These expressions, and others such as 'I did what I could' and 'This is all I could manage', fall between these two extremes. Success and failure are matters of judgement. To make such judgements, we often need to reflect on three fundamental questions:

- *What do I want to achieve?* This helps us focus on the change (if any) we wish to make, on how we would like things to be better and what would be regarded as a success. Having a clear and agreed view of how to achieve more success is vital.
- *What action can I take that might lead to greater success?* This is about being realistic and practical. I suggest it is also about working from an appreciation of your current strengths, gifts and talents. You might like to ask yourself 'What do I feel I can do myself, and what do I need help with?'
- *How will I know that something is a success?* This can be a bit tricky. Clearly not all change is a success. Also, things can change and your practice can get worse. So, not all change improves the existing situation. Sometimes things get worse before they get better. Much depends on the evidence used to make such judgements, like relative success or failure, and how the evidence is interpreted.

Illusions of prospection

Gilbert (2006) reminds us that we often suffer from 'illusions of prospection' when we ask ourselves questions such as 'What do I want to achieve?' When we ask this question, we try to work out what we want to aim for (e.g. 'better consistency of care within a multidisciplinary team') and what we want to avoid (e.g. 'unnecessary duplication of effort and resources'). Gilbert argues that when we look forward like this, we are prone to many of the illusions that bedevil our attempts to look outward ('outside the box') and backward (retrospective reflection-on-practice). He argues that we tend to overestimate the emotional consequences of future action. This is what is often called the 'impact bias'. There are several reasons for this. First, our imagination tends to make things up and leave things out. This means that the future we imagine can be quite different from the future we actually experience. Second, our current frame of mind, disposition, mood and so on, influence the way we imagine the future. Third, often we do not appreciate that the way we think about the future is not the way we think about it once it has happened. We have a tendency to overestimate how good we will feel when things go right and how bad we will feel when things go wrong. One way to try to understand how you will react emotionally to a future event or different way of working is to ask someone who has experienced, or is experiencing, this event. Gilbert (2006) suggests that one reason that we do not do this often enough is that we tend to regard ourselves as unique and that other people's experiences can't tell us much about how we might feel in the same situation. In this assumption, he suggests, we are wrong. People are not very different in their emotional reactions to events. The bottom line is that our predictions about the future, and our role in creating it, can lead us to make poor decisions. Gilbert argues persuasively that we tend to regret inaction more than action and that we do not feel as bad as we think we will if action leads to failure. This suggests that we should be more adventurous and more creative and take a few more risks. So, when asking yourself 'What do I want to achieve?' be bold!

Some kinds of reflection

More recently, there has been a developing appreciation that more than one kind of reflection exists. Table 1.4 shows four different kinds of reflection; each does a different job. In learning more about your work or workplace, and when trying to do something differently, you may have to be able to use more than one kind of reflection. In general, (a)–(d) in Table 1.4 can be done alone or with others, but (d) makes an explicit distinction between thinking alone and acting alone or in a workgroup/ team.

Really understanding reflection and the practices of it means you have to know something about Donald Schön's work. There is a huge amount written about Schön (Barnett 1997, Cossentino 2002, Eraut 1995, Parker 1997, Smyth 1991, Valkenburg & Dorst 1998). Schön (1983) wrote an important book called *The Reflective Practitioner*, with the subtitle *How Professionals Think in Action*. It is a book about the kinds of knowledge professionals need to do their job well. By implication then, it is a book about professional expertise. Schön talked about the importance of re-framing practice in order to make more sense of it (see p. 9). Re-framing means trying to see the same event from different viewpoints

Table 1.4 Kinds of reflection.

Reflection	Meanings
(a) Reflection-*in*-action	1. In a particular workplace
	2. Thinking on your feet, improvisation
(b) Reflection-*on*-practice	1. Before or after the event.
	2. On something significant
(c) Reflection-*for*-action	1. For a reason or particular purpose, e.g. improvement.
	2. Planning what you are going to do
(d) Reflection-*with*-action	1. Conscious future action.
	2. Action alone or with others

or perspectives in order to make more sense and deepen our appreciation of the event, for example re-framing a clinical event or encounter so we begin to see it freshly from the viewpoint of a child, parent, carer, nurse, doctor, physiotherapist, patient, and so on.

Schön developed the ideas of reflection-in-action and reflection-on-action. I have expanded each of these and suggest that we can think about these two notions like this:

- *Reflection-in-action:* This has two meanings. First, it means reflection in a particular context or workplace, for example in an office, on a ward, in a nursing home or in a hospital car park. Additionally, it can mean thinking about what you are doing while you are actually doing it. Some call this 'thinking on your feet'. Much of this can be unconscious. It's often called 'tacit knowledge'. For example, you ask a patient a question and then read the expression on her face; you see quickly that she doesn't understand what you have said, so you re-phrase the question in your mind and ask it again. This happens quickly, in the heat of the moment. So, reflection-in-action is about making on-the-spot adjustments to what you are doing, but in the midst of the action, not two or three days later. It is about improvisation and artistry (Eisner 1985).
- *Reflection-on-practice:* This also has two meanings. It can mean reflecting before or after the event, say a day or two later. This essentially involves looking back and going over things again. This kind of reflection is linked with the notion of time. It can also mean focusing on something significant. This may be part of a clinical 'encounter', an 'episode', a 'meeting', and so on. The hard thing is to ask yourself what is significant and what caught your eye and stayed in your memory. You could reflect on everything, but this is unwise, not healthy and often unnecessary.

Table 1.4 shows two further kinds of reflection:

- *Reflection-for-action:* This is fundamental. If you reflect on something you've done, been involved in or observed, presumably you are doing it for a particular reason. For example, you may want to understand it better, know more about it, change or improve it. These are all good reasons for reflecting on your work or that of others. This kind of reflection is also about planning to take some (positive) action to do something with what you've learned. This planning aspect is important because there is a difference between planning for action and action itself. For example, you might see and imagine something being different or better, but actually putting these thoughts into practice, in a particular workplace, is quite different. Additionally, for example, you might think of alternative ways of reducing the time a child waits to see a paediatrician. This is quite different from actually doing (or being able to do) something about reducing the wait time. Planning-for-action is sometimes called 'anticipatory reflection' (van Manen 1995).

- *Reflection-with-action:* This again has two meanings. First, it is actually about doing something. It is *conscious action* to develop your understanding or your skills. It is about weighing up what options you have, making a decision to act in a particular way, and then doing it. The 'with' part also means *acting alone or with others*. There are limits to learning and acting alone. Often, the power to change and improve something is achieved better by a group or team.

At this point I want to run an appreciative but more critical eye over some of the common assumptions we make about reflection before, during and after the event, and with regard to a particular kind of action – that which aims to improve something.

van Manen's view of reflective practice

van Manen (1999) stated that it is ironic that the attractive notion of reflective practice as 'retrospective reflection' or as 'anticipatory reflection' is unoriginal but likely, while the attractive idea of 'reflection-in-action' is original but unlikely. In other words, we might reflect on past and future actions to become more mindful, but to reflect on present actions while they unfold before us implies that we can step back from a clinical situation in order to consider what to say or do next. The attractive but problematic claim is that action, and reflection on this action, can be simultaneous. On the one hand, Schön argues that not only can we make the case that 'we can think about doing something but that we can think about something while doing it' (Schön 1983, p. 54). On the other hand, van Manen (1999) believes that reflection-in-action is compromised by at least two considerations: the relational structure of the interaction and the temporal dimensions of the practical contexts in which the action occurs. In other words, reflection-in-action is neither easy nor realistic. Reflecting on or about the experience of caring for a patient, performing an operation or making a home visit, and reflecting in the experience, are very different. Retrospective reflection on (past) experiences differs from anticipatory reflection on (future) experiences. In contrast, contemporaneous reflection in situations that permit a 'do, stop and think' kind of action differ markedly from more continuously dynamic clinical situations.

It seems, therefore, that there is a danger of overestimating the possibility of 'reflection-in-action, while acting' (van Manen 1994, 1995). Phenomenologically it is very difficult, if not impossible, for clinicians to be immersed in interactive activities with their clients/patients while simultaneously stepping back from the activity. On the other hand, some writers about reflection seem to underestimate the complexity of the organisation of basic everyday caring practice and the incredible intricacies of habitual practical actions in patient–professional encounters.

Berwick's view of reflective practice

What about the suggestion that reflection can be linked with improvements of one kind or another? Berwick (2004) argues that improvement is an inborn human endeavour. It takes no outside incentive. He also suggests that almost all human organisations contain, in their workforce, an internal demand to improve their work.

> It saddens me how few organisations seem to know that, and fewer still act on it. Improvement is not forcing something; it is releasing something.

(Berwick 2004, p. 1124)

But reflection with the intention to improve policy and practice, to improve the way healthcare organisations work, is not easy. The barriers and influences are many and can produce a sense of helplessness and futility. Often we may simply wish that someone, somewhere in the organisation, would give us that extra missing resource that would make change possible. 'We want to make care better,' goes the complaint, 'but they won't let us' (Berwick 2004, p. 1124).

Berwick (2004) links reflection for improvement with learning when he asks himself two positive questions. First, 'What is the story behind healthcare improvements in settings that have almost no slack?' Second, 'What are the assets that make improvement possible?' He reflects on successful improvement efforts in two challenging contexts, in Peru and Russia, and uncovers five types of asset that healthcare teams seem to use for leverage. In other words, he is saying that improvement can usefully begin with an appreciation and development of strengths. The assets are concerned with:

- consolidating aims for improvement;
- using team-based improvement projects in direct care settings;
- building infrastructure, especially human resources and data systems;
- altering the policy environment;
- spreading in stages.

Briefly, we can understand these assets thus:

Consolidating aims

Berwick (2004) states that clear aims provide an essential foundation for improvement in any setting. If you believe improvement is a planned process and rarely achieved by accident, then an organisation that wishes to improve must clearly formulate its intention to do so – its aims. This can be difficult. Setting specific targets that you have not accomplished before is a little frightening, especially if you lack an obvious process for getting there. In this book I suggest that you might usefully reflect on your successes and strengths and formulate your aims for further improvement around what you want more (not less) of. But the improvement aims have to fit well with what might be called a target-driven and results-oriented service. When reflecting for improved action, we need to be creative but also pragmatic.

Team-based improvement

The second major asset in the projects Berwick reviews is a bias towards 'teamness', the deeply held understanding that teams matter. He argues that resourceful teams find clever ways to do more with less.

Building infrastructure

The third asset is leaders being able to create local infrastructures in order to support improvement efforts.

Altering the policy environment

Local and pragmatic improvement efforts need politically astute people, agile at handling the wider policy environment.

Scaling up improvement

Berwick argues that this needs to be done in a step-by-step way, celebrating success, no matter how small, en route.

Later in the article, Berwick reflects on improvement processes: 'The lessons I am starting to learn from the people whose form of wealth is so different from mine' (Berwick 2004, p. 1128). He sets out a number of reflections. Here are nine of them, which, arguably, are transcontextual.

- *Simplify everything:* Improvement need not be complex. Set aims, track results, find great ideas, and change something every day to find the better ways. Involve everyone you can, and do not assume that the rules of today must be the rules of tomorrow. *Complexity is wasteful.*
- *Take teams seriously:* Improvement requires cooperation, and no one should trump the team. *Uncooperativeness is wasteful.*
- *Be pragmatic about measurement:* Numbers are useful. They can do certain kinds of job for us. Numbers, just like words, are open to interpretation. Use the least measuring that helps, not the most that you can think of. *Too much counting is wasteful.*

- *Strip the support system for improvement to a minimum:* Flatten the organisation. External consultants should make it their job to become unnecessary as fast as they can. *Dependency is a form of waste.*
- *Manage the political interface wisely:* It is wiser to know how to use it than to bang your head against it. *Naivety is wasteful.*
- *Help patients become advocates for change:* Their stake is the highest, and their voices count the most. *Keeping patients silent is wasteful.*
- *Go quickly. Start now:* Get on with an improvement initiative but only after a period of systematic reflection. Too much haste can create problems later. But *delay is wasteful.*
- *Make spread a system:* Find the latent structures, the channels along which change can flow, and use them from the start. *Isolation is wasteful.*
- *Don't complain:* Challenges and predicaments are all relative. There may always be some individual, group or organisation worse off than you right now. *Complaining is wasteful.*

(Berwick 2004, p. 1128)

Reflection and the complexities of practice

Many people think of reflective practice as if it was one 'thing' and that we do this 'thing' (the practice of reflection) in the same way. Also, for many years, reflective practice was thought to lead to the same outcome. This was about being a 'better' kind of person. 'Better' was generally about having more personal insight, more self-knowledge, more awareness and, for some, a greater ability to do something different. Another way of saying this is that it enabled the individual to change, or even improve, the way they saw themselves and how they acted in their world. This is a view of reflective practice that links the individual (e.g. a nurse) to an action (e.g. changing a patient's dressing) and this, in turn, with an outcome (e.g. an infection-free healthier patient). This view of reflective practice is shown in Fig. 1.2.

There is a danger if we leave these three links like this. The danger is around what's called 'linear thinking'. One thing leads to this, which leads on to that, and so on. Professional practice is messier and more complex than a description of it as 'three links'. There is also another

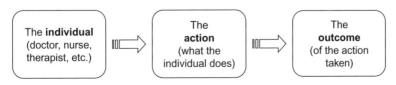

Figure 1.2   Simple three-link linear thinking.

important thing hidden behind this simple three-link description; this is concerned with assumptions. Here are some examples of the assumptions that Fig. 1.2 makes:

Assumption 1
The individual has a commitment and the ability and sees the need to reflect on what they do.
Assumption 2
The individual is able to act, in a particular way, at a particular time and in a certain workplace situation.
Assumption 3
The individual is clear about the choice of action (or inaction) being taken. Reflection-with-action (see Table 1.4) assumes that we are clear about a particular kind of action that we have in mind. But there are different kinds of action. We can usefully think about four kinds. They are:
- *Informed action:* This is about being clear about why you are acting (or not) in a particular manner. This kind of action is informed by your values.
- *Committed action:* This is being sure about what you are committed to doing.
- *Intentional action:* This is being clear about the purpose of your action (or inaction).
- *Sustainable action:* This is knowing how you can keep things going to achieve your intention(s).

Assumption 4
The individual can explain and justify the outcome of their action.
Assumption 5
If the outcome is 'good', then the individual might develop this into some kind of habit or routine that works for them.

These assumptions reveal some of the complexities of practice. But I wonder what might 'get in the way' to change, distort or improve the simple linear thinking shown in Fig. 1.2? What needs to be taken into consideration? What would Fig. 1.2 look like if we explicitly added seven more links to it? These links are:

- *Values:* How should I act?
- *Expectations:* What ought I to do?
- *Context:* What is actually possible here?
- *Decisions:* Is my action justifiable?
- *Reflection:* Could I have done anything better or different?
- *Judgement:* How far was this successful?
- *Intention:* What will I keep the same, or change, for next time?

You may like to try to re-draw Fig. 1.2 to insert these additional links. Where is the best place to insert them? How far does your re-drawn Fig. 1.2 still look simple and linear? How would you describe it now? What would happen if we stopped thinking about the individual and replaced it with *team* thinking? How does this affect your diagram? Team thinking is a move away from individual action to a consideration of collective action.

The centrality of the individual

Every act of reflection could invoke reflection on:

- *People:* Those involved in your practice, for example patients, clients, families and children.
- *How you, and they, feel and think:* What you feel affects how you think. This in turn affects what you do. The quality of your practice may be linked with how confident or inexperienced you feel when acting in a particular way.
- *Actions:* What it is you, and others, are actually doing, in a particular workplace. Any action requires a level of motivation. For example, you need to *want* to improve your practice.
- *Workplaces:* Workplaces have social, cultural and historical aspects.
- *Experiences:* That we and others have had. These may be positive or negative.
- *Your accountability:* This involves being able to describe, explain and then justify what you have (or have not) done.
- *Your values:* These are the things that make you the kind of person you are. They are important to you. They also give you reasons why you feel and think like you do. Values guide your practice (Ghaye 2005). Often they are quite hard to articulate. They may be about your personal or your working life. Sometimes it is not easy to draw a clear line between these two. Your values may be about being honest, sharing things, being fair, always trying to do your best, listening to and learning from others, and so on. Because our values are so important to us, the idea is that we should try to put them into practice. In other words, if you say you try to be honest with others, then you should not then act in a dishonest way. If fairness is one of your values, then you should try not to cheat. We cannot always put our values into practice, but we should try. When you are heard to say one thing but then do something else, you are a 'living contradiction' (Whitehead 2000). These contradictions in your practice are important things to reflect upon.

Reflective practices can be viewed as an *activity*. Schön (1983, 1987, 1991) wrote a lot about this. He argued that you should reflect on your everyday work, and especially anything that may be strange or puzzling about it. Reflective practices then become a *conscious activity*. Asking yourself questions such as 'What am I doing?', 'What happened?', 'What led to this?' and 'Why?' helps you reflect on, and learn more about, your work. If you do this regularly, and share your reflections with others, you give yourself opportunities to learn more about yourself, your strengths and your growth points.

Schön also said that reflection was a *critical activity*. If you ask 'How can I improve my practice?' you are questioning what you do, how you currently do things and the whole value of what you are doing. It involves questioning both ends and means. Asking fundamental questions such as this can help you think critically about why your practice was a success, failure or something in between. Being critical is *not* negatively pulling everything apart. It's more about trying to see things differently and do different things.

Dewey (1916, 1933) also wrote a lot about reflection. He said reflection was an *intentional activity*. The intention could be to pursue a planned course of action, to change or improve it. He argued that to do this successfully, you need the following three personal qualities:

- *Open-mindedness:* This is being receptive to the idea that improving your practice often means being open to new ideas.
- *Responsibility:* This is about being responsible for developing your personal and collective practice.
- *Wholeheartedness:* This is about how committed you are to continuously improve what you do. It's about giving things your best shot, at all times.

Arguably, reflective practices affect us. If you believe they do, then we should ask 'In what ways does knowledge, generated through the practices of reflection, affect us?' and 'How might these effects manifest themselves?' No one else can appreciate these effects unless we make a conscious and deliberate attempt to disclose them. O'Hanlon argues:

> ... reflection itself is invisible until the person takes action, and through that action e.g. a speech act, the person exposes his/her thoughts, perceptions, values and attitudes.

(O'Hanlon 1994, p. 283)

It is argued that reflective practices can also be a *creative activity*. Developing our competence is not simply thinking more and more about what we do. It is not about thinking harder and harder. Sometimes we have to think and act differently in order to improve our work. This can be a bit risky and can cause us to become anxious.

From reflective practice to practices

So what are we learning from all of this? One obvious thing is that 'reflective practice' should more accurately be the plural 'reflective practices'. The literature points to a complex array of meanings, methods and outcomes. We can also deduce that some view reflective practices as a way of linking intention (aims) with what is done (action) and its consequences (outcomes). Put another way, this is a view of reflective practices as action-oriented or action-orienting. A fundamental point is worth making about the relationship between reflection and action. You might reflect on yesterday's shift in the accident and emergency (A&E) department or on the signage (or lack of) in your hospital, without necessarily being 'oriented' to take any action. A central issue is whether you see reflection as part of the action or on the action. Dewey, regarded by some as one of the founding fathers of reflective practices, sees reflection as being directed towards action, namely the solving of a problem. So if he was confronted with a hospital way-finding problem (e.g. finding the outpatient department), he might ask an appropriate member of staff 'How do I get to the outpatient department from here?' In this way, the question is part of the action of solving the problem. For Dewey, reflection is a component of the action of solving the problem at hand. But this is not everyone's view. For example, some see reflective practices more as deliberations. Those that hold this basic view feel that there is no requirement that reflection must lead to action. Let us check we understand this point. Two frogs are sitting on a lily-pad. One decides to jump off. How many frogs are left? The answer is two, not one, because deciding is not the same as doing. We do not have to see the practices of reflection as pausing to take stock of a situation before we act (the same or differently), unless you are generally aligned with Dewey's view that reflection is prompted by an unsolved problem. We need to be open to the likelihood that we may, from time to time, want to get away from all life's problems in order to have an opportunity to reflect on other things.

Apart from the issues about the plurality of reflective practices and those about the relationship of reflection and action, there is one more thing the preceding pages help us appreciate. It is the impression generated by some literature in the field that critical forms of reflection are worthy, desirable and possible. I'm going to have a closer look at this now.

Some aspects of critical kinds of reflection

Ghaye (2005) argued that critical reflection was gaining popularity and tends to be caught up with terms such as 'emancipation', 'empowerment' and 'liberation'. The theoretical underpinning for it is generally offered by critical theory. This involves a look at the way in which history, identity construction, power, politics and different discourses, for example, affect the way we feel, think and act in particular settings. Increasingly, the practices of reflection have been informed by the 'critical being' movement (Brookfield 1995b, 2000a, 2000b, Carr & Kemmis 1986, Fay 1987, Rolfe *et al.* 2001). There are different versions of this movement in different disciplines, but Barnett (1997) suggests that there are three fundamental parts of the critical being: *critical thought*, *critical (self-)reflection* and *critical action*. Put another way, these are about particular kinds of self- and collective thinking and action. So what might critical reflection be? Rolfe *et al.* (2001)

hold Barnett's three ideas together when they define critical reflection as 'using the reflective process to look systematically and rigorously at our own practice.' They go on to say:

> We all reflect on our practice to some extent, but how often do we employ those reflections to learn from our actions, to challenge established theory and, most importantly, to make a real difference to our practice?

(Rolfe *et al.* 2001, p. i)

The ways of looking they outline are suggestive of a critical frame of mind, a general *critical disposition*. Barnett describes this as

> ... an ability to size up the world in its different manifestations and the capacity to respond in different ways ... the willingness to evaluate the world, howsoever it appears

(Barnett 1997, p. 87)

For me, this critical disposition also includes our ability to critique a body of knowledge and routine customs and practice. Some important related questions are:

- What is involved in critical consciousness? (Johns & Freshwater 1998)
- How can we avoid a situation of being reflective but thoroughly uncritical? (Barnett 1997)
- How can we remain critical and yet optimistic? (Brookfield 2000b)

Meaningful dialogue

It is worth mentioning that there are some powerful legacies of the idea of the critical being from Freire (1972, 1974, 1994, 1998). His emphasis on meaningful dialogue, on the process of problematisation and questioning the world, are highly relevant to improving healthcare today. A critical disposition helps to make us more aware that our practices could be other than they are. This disposition usually draws in big ideas such as (organisational) politics and ideology. These help us understand that the current state of play, in particular healthcare settings, is the result of historical and uneven forces.

> This ability to become critically conscious is far removed from simply examining an event to see what should be done differently. There is an implicit political dimension, linked to critical awareness, which enables assumptions inherent in ideologies to be challenged.

(Johns & Freshwater 1998, p. 152)

Kraft (1997, 2002) helps us appreciate that engaging in more critical (self)reflection brings with it the challenge of trying to respond positively to the consequences of such reflection, especially if it means having to make adjustments or changes to personal convictions or practices. This connection between critical reflection and the deliberate considera- tion of our own and others' values and (un)ethical conduct is also dis- cussed by Larrivee (2000) and Brookfield (1995a). Morley's work (2007) opens up another collection of appreciations about critical reflective practices.

Morley (2007) gives a reflective account of her practice with health practitioners who work as school nurses in the secondary education sys- tem in Victoria, Australia. She highlights some of the issues and dilemmas that emerged during her experiences, as a social work educator, facilitat- ing critical reflection workshops as a cross-disciplinary enterprise. Morley addresses two important questions: 'What are some of the difficulties and dilemmas in facilitating critical reflection workshops for school nurses as a social work educator?' and 'How can we use critical reflection to improve practice and education with professional colleagues who may have disciplinary backgrounds and values that may differ from our own?'

In contextualising her paper, the primary frameworks and perspectives Morley uses to understand and inform critical reflection are critical the- ories such as feminism (Clift 2005, Dominelli 2002, Marchant & Wearing 1986, Van Den Bergh & Cooper 1986), structural perspectives (Moreau 1979, Mullaly 1993, 2002), radical perspectives (Fook 1993) and critical postmodernism (Allan *et al.* 2003, Fook 1996, 2002, Hick *et al.* 2005, Ife 1997, Leonard 1997, Pease & Fook 1999). Interestingly, Morley conceptual- ises critical reflection in terms of a process or means of achieving the following three goals:

- *To improve practice:* Achieving this by promoting an analysis of the (in)congruencies between espoused values and values-in-action (Argyris & Schön 1976). She helpfully talks about critical values-in- action as, 'primarily concerned with practising in ways which further a society without domination, exploitation and oppression' focusing 'both on how structures dominate, but also on how people construct and are constructed by changing social structures and relations' (Fook 2002, p. 18). She argues that improving practice also includes 'Challenging our own self interests, and scrutinising how our own social positioning and implicit beliefs, values and assumptions may be complicit with inequitable social arrangements. This may take the form, for example, of examining how we understand, and possibly contribute to our own sense of powerlessness in certain contexts.'
- *To challenge and change dominant power relations and structures:* Her point here is that 'Using critical reflection can potentially liberate us from the way we construct structural problems and to reconstruct them in a way that emphasises our own personal agency.'
- *To create possibilities to practise critically in organisational contexts that are not necessarily conducive to critical practice:* Morley suggests that by

using a critical postmodern approach, the emancipatory possibilities for challenging, resisting and changing dominant power structures come within our grasp.

The critical reflection workshops for school nurses were part of an industry partnership between Deakin University and a major, local human service provider and lasted for 3.5 days. The workshop programme was based on the following principles and espoused the following aims:

- to introduce reflective practices to school nurses;
- to educate school nurses in the basic processes of critical reflection;
- to assist school nurses in the use of critical reflection as a personal process in evaluating their everyday work practices;
- to begin to develop, in a collaborative way and from actual practice experience, models for best practice in different contexts;
- to provide the basis for the healthcare organisation to use critical reflection in ongoing ways in the school nurse programme (Jones 2003).

So what did Morley learn? In an honest account, she examines:

- the school nurses' resistance to critical reflection;
- being perceived by the school nurses as being in cahoots with the nurses' management, and thus raising issues about trust between participants;
- confusion regarding the terminology of critical reflection;
- her own assumptions and constructions about each of these issues.

Questioning assumptions

Morley connects with Brookfield (1990), who explains:

> Questioning the assumptions on which we act and exploring alternative ideas is not only difficult but also psychologically explosive . . . Beginning to recognise and then critically question key assumptions is like laying down charges of psychological dynamite. When these assumptions explode and we realise that what we thought of as fixed ways of thinking and living are only options among a range of alternatives, the whole structure of our assumptive world crumbles. Hence, educators who foster transformative learning are rather like psychological and cultural demolition experts.

(Brookfield 1990, p. 178)

Brookfield also reminds us:

> In some cultures, people who think critically – who question accepted assumptions – are the first to disappear, to be tortured, or to be murdered in the event of a political *coup d'état*.

(Brookfield 1990, p. 179)

Not a pleasant thought. Therefore, in some organisations, engaging in critical reflection may be regarded as somewhat subversive, destabilising or threatening. As Tripp explains:

> We tend to set people up to accept and maintain a view of the world that is based on our own values; and because they are very valuable to us, very naturally we want those whom we teach to make our values their own.

(Tripp 1998, p. 36)

Critical action

So, critical reflection gets us thinking about critical action. But can action in, for example, the NHS in the UK be of this kind? Critical action is linked to our capacity to see ourselves in new ways and to do different things. Arguably critical action is about engaging in 'disruptive, sceptical and "other" social and discourse relations than those dominant, conventionalised and extant in particular fields' (Luke 2004, p. 26). In doing so, we need to be mindful of Brookfield's point that this might be energy-sapping, with staff leaving themselves 'feeling puny, alone, vulnerable and demoralised in the face of structural power that seems overwhelming and unchangeable' (Brookfield 2000b, p. 145). For critical action to happen, we need to find ways to step outside the frame of 'normal practices' and put on reflective lenses that help make the familiar and conventional, strange. This 'strangeness' might help us ask positive questions about practice, what it is like and how it has come to be the way it is. Critical action can be risky if done alone. It can lead quickly to stress and burnout. For staff who feel oppressed, marginalised and silenced, collective critical action might be a real way to try to move forward. Some of the important elements of critical action are:

- trying to lobby for and influence change;
- constantly holding under review (critiquing) our relationship with service structures and systems;
- engaging positively with forms of political oppression and repression in the places where we work, and particularly in debates about who gets what, where and how.

Linking reflection with learning and practice

Learning is about the way we acquire knowledge, skills and sensitivities. Learning is about expanding what we know, extending what we are able to do and enriching how we feel. Learning also involves making sense of ideas and actions, and organising and 'managing' them. Some learning helps us understand a situation better. Other learning is 'put to work'. We apply it to something. This means we actually do something with what we know.

Reflective practices help us with four kinds of learning. They are:

- *Cognitive learning:* Helping us think about things differently, perhaps more creatively.
- *Affective learning:* Helping us learn through feeling and emotion.
- *Action learning:* Helping us turn what we think and feel into ethically literate and responsible actions.
- *Social learning:* Helping us learn from and with others.

If you want to demonstrate developments in your practice, you might usefully reflect upon the following six things:

- Where you are now: this is knowing the strengths and limitations of your current practice.
- What you need to keep doing well.
- The areas in which you need to improve.
- How best to move forward.
- How to learn from success, no matter how small.
- What the evidence of positive development looks like, and how far it will be accepted as valid.

To develop your practice, you may need at least four kinds of knowledge. They are:

- *Personal knowledge* gained when in work (on the job) and for work, gained while thinking about what you have done or could do.
- *Collective knowledge* gained by working with others, both in and out of the workplace.
- *Practical knowledge* gained by reflecting on what works best and what works less well for you, in particular settings.
- *Public knowledge* gained by accessing the recorded experiences of others, published and available online, in journals and books.

Some senior managers ask me bluntly: 'Will reflection lead to better practice and better services for our patients/clients?' Any time invested in reflective practices needs to be time well spent. So how can this happen in practice? Here are five things to think about:

- being in the right frame of mind;
- using a structured process;
- support at the right time;
- conversations with significant others (e.g. tutor, mentor, coach, supervisor);
- time, resources and the opportunity to do it.

Sometimes we find ourselves in a frame of mind where it feels like we cannot do anything more, or different, in order to improve our practice. We feel stuck. Sometimes this is due to genuine humility or self-doubt. Sometimes we feel we do not have enough energy to make the extra effort that continuously developing our practice requires. Feeling stuck and going nowhere is not pleasant. It is important to be aware of feelings like these and to try to create opportunities to discuss them in a reflective conversation with trusted others. As mentioned earlier, fear can also get in the way of developing your practice. It may be a fear that your proposed improvement will be a failure (real or imagined) and that you might end up being blamed for things going wrong.

Additionally, you could spend some time thinking about the following three 'P's and what they really mean to you. Reflecting on the three 'P's means you:

- *Reflect on your passions:* Nothing motivates us more than our passions in life. Our passions get us going like nothing else. In your working life, what are you passionate about? What do you love to do? A passion is something you care about a lot. If you focus on your passions, your practice is likely to grow in that direction.
- *Reflect on your proficiencies:* What are you good at doing? Everyone has gifts and talents. What are your strengths, *as perceived by you*, and in particular work settings? To develop your practice, you need to know what you really love to do and what you really want to be good at doing. These can be tough decisions, because they mean you need to align your passions with your performance.
- *Reflect on your priorities:* Working on what you love to do requires you to focus on your passions. Getting better at what you love to do means you have to be able to prioritise. You have to identify what's important to get better at, prioritise these things and then actualise, or do something about each one. Reflecting carefully on your work, who you are working with and where makes prioritising easier. You should think about what you need to do immediately and what you can leave until later. Another consideration is making a distinction between what you feel is important to you to develop and what others feel you should work at developing. You may also need to think about the difference between what you feel you could do and must do. The more specific we can be, the more likely we are to be successful in developing our practice.

Linking reflection with good practice

Developing our practice means that we are developing the quality of our work. High-quality work is at the heart of good practice. Because our competence is about our ability to do things, it is therefore about performance and achievement. This may be on a personal or collective (workgroup, team, organisational) level. But how you do what you do is about ethics. Who wants to work with a high performer who is like this only because of the way they use, exploit, disempower and silence anyone who may threaten or challenge their supremacy? Given a choice, who wants to

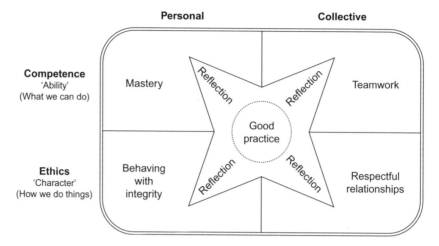

Figure 1.3   Linking reflection with good practice.

work with a high achiever who cheats and lies their way to the top and is clever enough to avoid getting caught? Ethics is, therefore, about how we behave. This is linked to our personal qualities or character.

Figure 1.3 shows how competence (what we can do) and ethics (how we do things), at both a personal and a collective level, are linked. It also shows the links between these and reflection. It is important to note that reflection is not 'added on to' practice, like an afterthought. It is embedded *in* practice.

What are some of the habits of reflection?

So how might we go on to think about reflecting on something significant? One possibility is to think about how far you could make the practices of reflection a *work habit*. Here are five possible habits of reflection:

Habit 1   **Reflecting on your values**
These guide everything you do. They are your reasons for doing this and not doing that. This should become a *conscious habit*.

Habit 2   **Reflecting on your feelings**
This can be painful, so it is important to make sure you have some support when you do this. This should be a *supported habit*.

Habit 3   **Reflecting on your thinking**
This can open up options for future action. This is best done through conversation with others. There are limits to thinking alone. This should be a *collegial habit*.

Habit 4   **Reflecting on your actions**
This is essential if we are ever to improve what we do. Much can be gained if this is done collectively with some of those who witnessed your action. This is a *collaborative habit*.

Habit 5 **Reflecting on context**
Reflecting on all the above is one thing. Reflecting on the workplace context in which they are all embedded is something else. This habit requires holistic thinking. This is the habit that enables us to understand that what we do is always context-dependent. The context in which we work serves to constrain or liberate us. It allows and encourages us to do things. It can also suffocate, frustrate and disempower us. This is a *political habit*.

Some frameworks for action

There are many models of reflection. You can find examples and a critique of some of them in Ghaye & Lillyman (2006a). Initially, most people like some kind of guidance and structure to help them reflect in a systematic and useful way. Using a model can help with this. But we should not think that using a model will suit us perfectly. We may find some models more appealing than others, some easier to use or understand than others. We need to be careful about becoming a slave to any one model. Also, we need to be on our guard if we begin to feel that using a particular kind of model is reducing reflection to a simple, orderly forward-stepping process. Thinking and learning are often messy and with lots of 'unfinished business'. They are not often linear either. We may go forward, and then feel we are going backwards. We may make rapid progress and then get stuck. Going forward is not always wise. Sometimes it is better to take a step back, re-think and then go forward again, but this time differently.

Schön (1983, 1987) did not use the word 'model' but chose the phrase 'frame for action'. I briefly illustrate four kinds of frame to further develop an appreciation of some important features on this 'rough ground'. There are some similarities in the content of each one. There are those that frame thinking and action around:

- questions
- stages
- levels
- cycles.

Questions first. Johns (2006) offers a 'model for structured reflection'. He calls questions 'reflective cues'. Some examples are:

- Focus on a description of an experience that seems significant in some way.
- What is the background of this experience?
- What particular issues seem significant to pay attention to?
- How do I interpret the way others were feeling and why they felt that way?
- How was I feeling, and what made me feel that way?

There are also some frames organised around the idea of stages. Boyd & Fales (1983) suggest six stages. Stages are about moving from one to another. They imply an orderly sequence. Their first stage begins with a sense of inner discomfort. Their sixth stage is a consideration of whether to act on the outcome of the reflective practices.

King and Kitchener's (1994) reflective judgement model also suggests that a learner passes through various stages of reflection. These stages are the pre-reflective, quasi-reflective and reflective thinking stage. In the pre-reflective phase, knowledge is first limited to simple, concrete observations about what we think is true. This then starts to develop into knowledge being either absolutely certain or temporarily uncertain. In the quasi-reflective stage, we would begin to understand that knowledge can be uncertain and that some problems are not solved easily. We would be able to use evidence but might have difficulty justifying our beliefs and drawing reasoned conclusions. Finally, in the reflective thinking stage, we see knowledge not as fixed and given but as a means of reasoned enquiry and problem-solving. Solutions and judgements are based on data and enquiry. But we appreciate that these can always be re-evaluated in the light of new evidence.

The frame Larrivee (2000) developed is in three stages. The process of becoming a reflective practitioner weaves through these, the first of which is the *examination* stage. At this stage we start to question whether a particular action, reaction or interaction is getting us what we want. It could be any behaviour that we are bringing into question, such as getting angry, engaging in power struggles or withdrawing. In stage 1 Larrivee (2000) suggests we begin to notice patterns in our ways of behaving and challenge the real cost attached to our current practice. We come to realise that our behaviour is sustaining a state we want to change.

Attempting to let go of what is familiar leads us into stage 2 – *struggle*. Here we can find ourselves in all sorts of conflict. This begins a significant stage in the reflective process. If this state of inner turmoil brings about too much fear and doubt, then the choice may be to close down the process and either stay with the old practice or seek a quick fix. We look for a ready-made solution, a prescription for change. Working positively through stage 2 provides us with an opportunity to make a *perceptual shift* (stage 3), where new discoveries lead to a transformation of current practice.

Moving on to levels, Mezirow's (1981) levels of reflection (or, more correctly, 'levels of consciousness') are about an increasing 'depth of reflection'. His two levels are called the consciousness and critical consciousness levels. The first level embraces reflections on how we feel, perceive relationships between things and become aware of how we make value judgements. The latter concerns reflections on personal prejudices and context.

Into cycles: there are many frames of this kind. A popular one is that of Gibbs (1988). It begins by asking you to describe what happened.

It also has a feelings element. This is important because reflection is often triggered by feelings. A detailed illumination of this can be found in Ghaye & Lillyman (2006a).

Kolb & Fry (1975) formulated a learning cycle (or, more precisely, a learning spiral) with four elements: concrete experience, observation and reflection, the formation of abstract concepts, and testing in new situations. They suggest that the learning cycle can begin at any one of the four points. For many people, the cycle usually begins with a person actually doing something (with an action) and then some reflections on the effect or impact of the action on the people or things involved.

The reflective practitioner

Donald Schön's (1983) notion of the reflective practitioner is very popular. His focus of attention was essentially on the way individuals acted at work. He celebrated the ability and motivation individuals had to understand themselves better and to improve themselves and their work. He said we needed 'practical knowledge' in order to do this. Schön had an optimistic vision of the power of individuals to change. He believed them to be adaptive and intentional people, willing and perhaps able to better understand their work and improve what they did. His views are linked closely with the notion of self-reflection. They are aligned with a culture of individualism, which this book moves away from in steps 2 and 3.

In his classic book *The Reflective Turn*, Schön (1991) encourages practitioners to ask some fundamental questions about their work, particularly if their practice is puzzling or strange in some way. In Schön's work we find four serious questions, namely:

- What do practitioners/learners need to know?
- What is it appropriate to reflect upon?
- What is an appropriate way of observing and reflecting on practice?
- How would we know if this has been done rigorously?

Schön argued that reflective practitioners asked themselves these questions. They not only learned from reflection but also responded appropriately to events and situations as they experienced them.

As mentioned earlier, Schön's work celebrated the experiential learning of practitioners in everyday action. He called this learning in the 'swampy lowlands' of actual practice. Swampy lowlands are actual workplaces wherein lie the problems of greatest human concern and where messy, confusing problems defy a simple technical solution. Critical reflection, says Schön, is more than simply reflecting-in or reflecting-on action. When you engage in critical reflection you question the way you 'frame' or 'see' the problems of practice in the first place. Even if no apparent problems exist, as a critically reflective practitioner you would question situations, asking why things are they way they are and why events unfold in the way they do. Critical reflection, according to Schön, involves questioning what you might routinely take for granted. When you reflect critically on your own practice, you problematise your own actions, asking questions such as 'Why did I do that?', 'What values inform my practice?' and 'How are these values helping or hindering my work?'

The work of Dewey

John Dewey (1933) argued that reflective processes cannot be separated from some sort of event called an 'experience'. It follows that reflective practitioners use 'experience' as their raw material for learning. He also emphasised that not all experience educates. For example, can you remember living through events from which you emerged (apparently) unchanged? Have you ever felt that you have missed out and not learned lessons that others have learned, having gone through the same experience as you? Dewey wrote that in order for learning to happen, an experience must include two key elements. The first is continuity. This means that to learn something, you need to be able to connect aspects of the new experience to what you already know. This may add to what you already know. It may modify or improve it. The second element is interaction. This means that in order to learn something you need to be actively interacting with others in your workplace, continuously testing out and modifying what you are learning in the company of others. Dewey (1933) also argued that reflective practitioners learn by noticing and framing problems of interest in particular ways. He said that if you experience surprise or discomfort in your everyday work, then the reflective process is triggered.

Dewey's notion of a 'problem'

Loughran (2006) develops Dewey's notion of a 'problem'. He warns that although reflecting on problems is important, it should not be done at the expense of other aspects of our working life. He also states that using the word 'problem' has negative connotations and conjures up images of mistakes and errors of judgement. Loughran re-defines a problem as:

> . . . a situation that attracts attention; something that is curious or puzzling; something that invites further consideration beyond that which might initially have been anticipated.

(Loughran 2006, p. 45)

Dewey saw reflective thinking as a way to discover specific connections between actions and consequences. He believed that reflective thinking would help you learn from your experience and improve your problem-solving skills.

Further, Dewey argued that the reflective process consisted of several steps, including: (i) 'perplexity, confusion, doubt' due to the nature of the situation in which one finds oneself; (ii) 'conjectural anticipation and tentative interpretation' of given elements or meanings of the situation and their possible consequences; (iii) 'examination, inspection, exploration, analysis of all attainable considerations', which may define and clarify a problem with which one is confronted; (iv) 'elaboration of the tentative hypothesis suggestions'; and (v) deciding on 'a plan of action' or 'doing something' about a desired result (Dewey 1973, pp. 494–506). van Manen (1995) argues that a proper sequencing of such reflective steps makes up reflective experience, which in turn can lead to analysis and evaluation, and then to further reflective action.

The work of Habermas

Jurgen Habermas (1974), like Dewey, also had plenty to say about reflection and experience. He saw reflective practices as a way of questioning experience and, in so doing, freeing the mind from unchallenged assumptions. He also saw reflection as a kind of investigatory process that has the potential to lead to personal enlightenment and emancipation. His work is also aligned with Schön in the sense that he believed that knowledge is sought on the basis of self-interest.

> Yet in making the connection to action, Habermas did not see that knowledge generated by individual (critical) reflection was in itself sufficient for social action. He believed it was necessary to engage in discursive processes through which participants in the situation came to an authentic understanding of their situation.

(O'Hanlon 1994, p. 285)

I'll pick up on this point about discussion (or the importance of certain kinds of conversation) in action step 3 (see p. 161).

The work of Mezirow

Jack Mezirow (1978, 1990) presented a theory of transformative learning whereby reflection on experience, and particularly critical reflection, is central. Mezirow's theory of 'transformative learning' is based on a three-level view of critical reflection on experience. Mezirow suggests that when we encounter a 'disorienting dilemma', a problem for which there is no immediately apparent solution suggested by our past experience and knowledge, reflection is often triggered. In such circumstances, he suggests, we tend to reflect first on the content of the experience; this is on 'what happened'. If we find and test a solution to the problem that produces undesirable outcomes, then we move to a second level. Here, we usually reflect on the process (e.g. how we were doing something). We ask ourselves questions such as 'How did it happen that way?' A third level is reached if we reflect upon the foundation (e.g. deep-seated values and assumptions) guiding our work. In this third level of reflection, we confront and challenge our taken-for-granted ways of working.

We ask ourselves questions such as 'What's wrong with what I did and how it happened?' Mezirow argued that level-three reflection leads to a dramatic shift or transformation in the way we view what we are doing. Mezirow (1990, p. 29) describes this process of transformative learning as the 'bringing of one's assumptions, premises, criteria, and schemata into consciousness and vigorously critiquing them'.

The work of Zeichner & Liston

Zeichner & Liston (1996) say that reflective practitioners examine, re-frame and attempt to solve the 'dilemmas of practice'. Reflective practitioners can do this because they are:

- aware of and question the assumptions and values they bring to their work;
- attentive to the institutional and cultural contexts in which they work;
- involved in workplace change efforts;
- able to take responsibility for their own professional development.

The work of Day

Chris Day (1999) offers another thought that is essentially about improving practice by gaining a sense of perspective on things. He states that the reflective practitioner is:

> . . . one who, given particular circumstances, is able to distance herself from the world in which she is an everyday participant and open herself to influence by others, believing that this distancing is an essential first step towards improvement.

(Day 1999, p. 218)

What Day embraces here is the idea that reflection is for the improvement of practice. He also leaves the door open for us to think about the different ways we might create this 'distance'. One way is to engage in some personal reflection, after the event, and in a solitary manner. Another is to do this in a small group, more publicly and through conversation.

The work of Pollard

Andrew Pollard (2002, 2005) makes a clear link between the reflective practitioner and reflective teaching – in other words, what teachers do. Reflective nursing would be what nurses do, and so on. Pollard's seven characteristics of the actions of reflective practitioners are:

- having an active concern with both the aims of practice and the consequences of it. This is what Pollard calls an interest in 'moral purpose'. It is reflective practices that are about making a positive difference to the learning and lives of others;

- engaging in a cyclical process of continuous monitoring, evaluation and revisions of the practitioner's own work;
- demonstrating informed judgements that result from being competent in the methods of evidence-based workplace enquiry;
- being open-minded, responsible and wholehearted (see Dewey's work);
- having an ability to draw upon and actively use ideas and views from research;
- collaboration and dialogue with colleagues;
- creatively linking a practitioner's understanding of their own values, in their own workplace, with any external professional body and government requirements.

Why are reflective practices important?

There are many books that set this out (Bulman 2004, Ghaye 2005, Jasper 2007, Johns 2006). In summary, there are at least three answers to this question:

- *Personal importance:* Reflection helps develop our self-awareness, self-knowledge and self-belief. Developing these can help us do our best at all times.
- *Professional importance:* Reflection can help us develop our competence. In other words, it is important because it helps us continuously improve what we do and for whom.
- *Political importance:* It is hard to argue that we work in isolation. It is realistic to argue that we work in a 'context'. Our work is always in a social and cultural context: a social context, as in a workgroup or team, and in a cultural context, as in a supportive workplace or with people of different ages, experiences, values and beliefs. We always work in an historical context in the sense that we probably worked 'there' yesterday and today. This can influence what we do 'there' tomorrow. We also work in a political context. By this, I mean that reflective practices can help us understand local workplace politics. This is about who gets what, when and how in our workplace. It helps us understand what we should do. These must-dos are often written down in policy documents, curricula, protocols and programmes of study. Reflection helps us understand who gets on with whom, who has power and influence, who gets things done, who needs persuading if you want something, and so on.

Reflective practice in medical education

Interestingly, there has been a growing awareness of the importance (and need) for the practices of reflection in medical education. This has no doubt been spurred on in the UK by the government's modernising medical careers initiative and the new two-year postgraduate foundation

Table 1.5 The importance of reflective practices in the education of tomorrow's doctors.

Question	Evidence base
Why are reflective practices important in medical education?	Albanese (2006): crucial for all doctors in the UK for the processes of appraisal and revalidation, for lifelong learning (policy imperative)
	Mamede & Schmidt (2004): reflecting consciously upon one's own professional practice is important for the development of expertise (professional imperative)
	Sobral (2000): enables medical students to obtain greater benefit and enjoyment from their studies, greater readiness for application, change in behaviours and commitment to action (personal imperative)
What are some of the positive outcomes of this?	Fish & de Cossart (2006): helps develop the essence of medical practice, decision-making and sound judgement
	Bleakley (2002): moves education from a transmission model to a student being actively involved in their own learning
	Rider & Brashers (2006): development of teamwork and ability to work effectively in multidisciplinary teams
	Zebrack & Fletcher (2006): can capture learning in-the-moment

curriculum for junior doctors. Table 1.5 summarises some of the developments in this area.

Getting organised for engaging in reflective practices

Reynolds & Vince (2004) make an important point that links directly with the central question I raised in the introduction: that less time needs to be spent on reflection as something we do, as an individual, and more time given to creating opportunities for us to reflect with others. Reynolds and Vince say this can be done only if organisations become better organised for supporting reflective practices. Table 1.6 sets out eight general things to think about in getting organised for reflection.

Table 1.6 Eight things to think about in getting organised for reflection.

Think	Question
You	Will you do it alone or within a group or team?
Level	Where will it be done within your organisation? In a department, clinic, unit, curriculum subject area, etc.?
Motive/s	Why do you want to try to learn through reflective practices?
Right/s	How far do you have time that is protected to reflect on your practice?
Rules	How can you get organised so that you can get the most from the practices of reflection?
Resources	What resources do you need in order to engage productively in reflective practices?
Impact	How far do you want (or need) to demonstrate a real and worthwhile outcome from doing reflective practices?
Ethics	How far do you feel reflective practices will help you act ethically? This is about enabling you to understand the reasons why you do things, the way you treat others and how they interact with you.

Reflective practices and workplace cultures

A workplace is a complex environment. There are some important qualities that will make it a real 'learning environment'. It is important to be aware of the things that are likely to support workplace learning and what might get in the way. In every workplace there are people who understand the practices of reflection and are able to support you to learn through them. But there are also others who misunderstand the nature, processes and outcomes of reflective practices and may even be sceptical and hostile towards them. Table 1.7 shows four basic attitudes people might display towards reflective practices in your workplace.

Reflective practices and trust

Learning through reflection needs to be a supported process. It is important that we seek out colleagues and peers with the attitudes described in the I can/I will box. Clearly the people to be avoided (if possible) are those in the I can't/I won't box, who make it obvious that they can't support you, and, even if they could, wouldn't support you.

Learning through reflective practices, in any context, is dependent upon trust. Trust affects the way we interact with others. It influences how we feel and what we say and do. Maister *et al.* (2002) offer six aspects of trust.

Table 1.7   Attitudes towards reflective practices in the workplace.

	I will	**I won't**
I can	I can, and I am willing to support you	I can but I won't because . . .
I can't	I can't right now, but I am willing to support you in principle	I can't, and even if I could I wouldn't because . . .

All of them are important, especially when discussing topics such as what you have learned, what you might do differently next time and why people act in the ways they do. Trust is also a vital part of a helpful and fulfilling after-work 'reflective conversation' with someone more experienced than you (e.g. a tutor). The aspects are:

- *Trust grows:* It doesn't happen by magic. We may have to work at it.
- *Trust is emotional:* Knowing we can trust someone helps us feel good. If this trust is broken, it can be upsetting.
- *Trust is a two-way relationship:* We won't get the most from reflective practice unless we find people who we trust, people with whom we can speak openly and honestly. They need to respect our openness and honesty and not abuse it.
- *Trust involves risk:* Who we learn to trust and what we trust them with can be a risky business. Without a real trusting relationship with significant others (e.g. tutor, mentor, coach, supervisor), our reflections may stay 'safe' and predictable. We may not feel we can get to the real issues that are on our mind.
- *Trust is experienced differently:* On balance, we might feel we can trust ourselves to say and do the 'right' thing at the 'right' time. But how far would others hold the same view of us? We may feel we cannot trust someone. How far do you think others feel the same way?
- *Trust is personal:* Who can you really trust with your feelings and thoughts? It might be useful to try to aspire to what follows when choosing to share your reflections with others. 'I know I can trust you to do the best you can for me. You can trust me to play my part in this learning process and I understand that our reflective conversations are based on this shared value.'

Attitudes towards reflection

Ultimately, only you can be responsible for your own learning through reflection. Others can help and support you, but it is you and your attitude to learning that matter most. Here are six attitudes to try to avoid:

- *Being passive:* This means you don't act positively in situations that need action.

- *Being helpless:* There is usually something that you can do to improve your practice. The key is thinking about what you can practically do, in the circumstances. It's about knowing what is, and is not, in your control.
- *Disabling self-talk:* You should avoid talking yourself out of things. If you hear yourself constantly saying 'I can't do it' or 'It won't work', seek help.
- *Being caught up in a negative spiral:* Sometimes one setback can lead to a succession of negative thoughts. A plan doesn't go well. You then lose a sense of self-worth. You lose heart and confidence and everything feels like it is spiralling downwards, maybe towards inaction. If you feel this way, seek help.
- *Feeling that you can't be bothered:* This is a very negative thought. You should ask yourself 'Why am I feeling like this?' 'Is it boredom?' 'Have I lost interest in what I am doing?' 'Did I begin with enthusiasm but have learned some lessons that have made work tedious?' If you feel this way, you have to decide whether you wish to seek help.
- *Choosing not to change:* Learning often requires that you do things differently. You may also have to do different things. You may feel you have the right to choose not to change. But what is the price of this? What are the consequences of not changing?

Learning in the clinical environment: the work of Hart & Rotem

Hart & Rotem (1995) asked 516 registered and student nurses questions about how they perceived professional development while working in clinical settings. They found some positive correlations between professional development and six aspects of the cultures in a variety of clinical areas. They also found that some wards and hospital environments supported learning better than others. The six aspects are:

- *Autonomy and recognition:* The extent to which we feel valued and are encouraged to take responsibility for our own practice.
- *Job satisfaction:* The extent to which we enjoy working in the place.
- *Role clarity:* The extent to which we understand what is expected of us.
- *Quality of supervision:* The extent to which we are given practical advice and support from more experienced staff.
- *Peer support:* The extent to which those we are working alongside are friendly, caring and supportive towards one another.
- *Opportunities for learning:* The extent to which meaningful opportunities to learn, grow and improve are available.

This research has big implications for learning through reflective practices. Ideally, everything is required, in the workplace, if we are to get the most from reflective learning. For example, if you are encouraged to take responsibility for your own practice, then you are more likely to be asking yourself important reflective questions such as 'How can I sustain my best practice?' and 'How can I improve what I am doing here?' If the quality of supervision and peer support is high, then you are likely to be more able to share what you are really thinking and feeling. If there are real opportunities to do this, then there is a chance that you will continue to learn and grow.

Workplace learning for nurses, accountants and engineers: the work of Eraut et al.

The funded project of Eraut *et al.* (2004) comprised:

- a longitudinal study of the learning of 30 nurses, 30 accountants and 30 engineers at the start of their careers;
- a study of the transition from higher education into employment, in relation to technical knowledge and generic skills.

The three professions were chosen because they play key roles in the UK economy and public services and because they use contrasting approaches to professional development. The employers of graduate accountants and engineers have systems of organised training support. The newly qualified, post-diploma nurses in the project started full-time work with greater practical experience than accountants or engineers.

Eraut *et al.* (2004) found that there were six factors that affected early career workplace learning. These factors were not always 'experienced' in the same way by those in each profession. Their general findings were grouped as learning and as contextual factors.

Learning factors

All of these factors are linked. Eraut *et al.* (2004) argue that confidence, challenge and support are linked like this. Learning at work requires confidence and this, in turn, is linked with the extent to which 'workers' are able to successfully meet work challenges. The confidence to take on these challenges depends upon the extent to which workers feel supported in doing this. Additionally, feedback, value and commitment are linked like this. Feedback is vital in early career learning as a check on progress and personal development. It can be seen as a form of support. The value of the work being done is a positive force and enhances individual commitment to learning. They conclude:

> . . . both confidence in one's ability to do the work and commitment to the importance of that work are primary factors that affect individual learning.

(Eraut *et al.* 2004, p. 8)

Contextual factors

Again these are linked in some important ways. For example, the allocation and structuring of work are central to workers' career progress.

This affects who is encountered at work and in what ways, for example whether it is individual work or teamwork. Progress is not only something a worker needs to feel but is also linked with the expectations others have of them.

An appreciative framework for supporting the learning of teams of health and social care workers: the work of Ghaye (2005)

From work with 753 teams of health and social care workers during the period 1999–2004, I was able to develop an evidence-based, appreciative framework for supporting reflection in the workplace. This is shown in Fig. 1.4.

The development of the framework has generally been influenced by a commitment to positive, people-centred approaches to organisation, team and individual improvement. Much of the spirit of this work is captured by the art and practice of appreciative enquiry (Cooperrider & Whitney 2005). The framework seeks fundamentally to build a constructive union between individuals and workgroups/teams on the one hand and their capabilities to create more possible and improved futures on the other hand. Figure 1.4 shows that the framework is constructed around ten attributes. These are organised into three zones. Each zone is a source for positive change. Care, creativity and improvement form the positive core of values and practices.

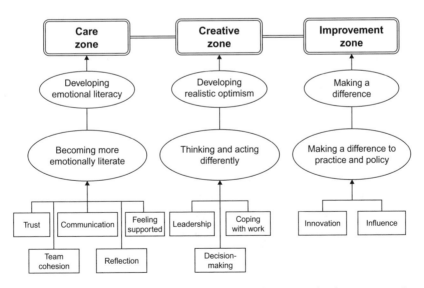

Figure 1.4 Evidence-based appreciative framework for supporting reflective team-based learning.
(After Ghaye 2005)

One of the fundamental appreciations from the framework is this: in order to learn in the workplace, thus improving what we do with and for others, we need to attend to those things in the 'care zone'. These attributes are all about getting relationships 'right'. If these things are as good as they can or need to be, it gives us the confidence to try to think and act differently. This involves working with the attributes in the 'creative zone'. In turn, this provides a sound platform for trying to improve individual or collective practice, maybe develop policy and 'make a difference'. This involves those attributes in the 'improvement zone'. So there is a developmental learning story that runs left to right on Fig. 1.4.

Sometimes the storyline goes the other way, from right to left. For example, you might find that you are working in a healthcare organisation where your colleagues are being made redundant, recruitment of new staff is frozen and hospital admissions are increasing. This requires you instantly to change and improve what you do. Now working from right to left in Fig. 1.4 is important. For example, in this scenario, you may need to make some bold and different decisions. You may have to be creative. New leadership may also be needed. All this impacts on existing patterns of working relationships. These may also have to change. So you may have to look again at your 'care zone' attributes. This oscillation back and forth (right to left, and vice versa) is an acknowledgement of both the challenges of practice and of service improvement.

In many workplaces, the dominant culture is one of doing, with little time for reflection and, therefore, workplace learning. Perhaps we need to be better about linking 'cultures of doing' with cultures of 'learning while doing'. Organisational improvement begins with individuals. Unless we can demonstrate that we can improve our practice, there can be no meaningful team or organisational improvement. If *we* can't change, then organisations cannot change either.

Re-framing reflective practices

Here in action step 1 we begin our journey across the rough ground I described in the introduction. Initially I suggested that this might be regarded (by some readers) as relatively familiar terrain. Now the ground may become less familiar, rougher, as I re-frame the purposes and practices of reflection in the light of what we currently know. My reason for this is to get us into a position to understand how we may have to re-frame reflective practices if we are to try to scale them up to become organisation-wide work habits.

Developing the reflective healthcare team

In *Developing the Reflective Healthcare Team*, I set out what I called the 'four interests of reflective practice' (Ghaye 2005, pp. 47–91). In that book, my systematic review of what appeared to be the preoccupations of those in the field looked like this:

Interest 1: being human well

This embraced reflections on personal wellbeing and being human well. I described this interest as essentially being about self-reflection and associated more broadly with a view of the humanity of the person, which is infused by self-understandings (Watson 1999). It casts the role of the practices of reflection as developing a heightened sense of one's being. These might be developed alone or through interaction and dialogue with others. This interest was unsurprisingly aligned with Schön's (1983) work on the reflective practitioner and in some more contemporary writing, for example in the area of reflective self-study (Freshwater 2002, Higgs & Andresen 2001, Johns 2001, 2002, 2004, Johns & Freshwater 1998, McCormack 2001, Stuart 2001).

Interest 2: embracing uncertainty

This was described as using the practices of reflection to help us make sense of our work, working life and workplaces. It was an interest that seemed particularly relevant in the context of healthcare reform and workplace transformation. It was about the work of those who used reflective practices in a context of endemic uncertainty, complexity, short planning horizons, financial stringency, different and greater stakeholder involvement. This interest was aligned with the work of Dewey (1933). More theoretically, the interest was underpinned by the early work of Gleick (1991) on 'chaos', Stewart & Golubitsky (1992) on 'complexity' and Stewart (1995) on 'order and pattern'.

Interest 3: the bottom line

This was all about reflective practices serving individual and collective interests to improve practice, meet targets and get better results. It was linked with concrete and tangible outcomes that were 'good' not only for the individual healthcare worker but also for a service, for users of those services and thus for the organisation. It was associated with much of the current management-speak about eradicating waste, adding value and serving 'customer needs'. It was about getting more from the same, or less, about applying lean principles, balanced scorecards, value streams, benchmarking, and so on. These all tend to go in and out of vogue, but benchmarking

> ... is most definitely back to centre stage as healthcare organisations wrestle with the quest to become even more efficient. Central to this is how does a hospital or general practice compare with its peer group?

(Amos 2006, p. 32)

An interest in the bottom line is an interest in how much 'discretionary effort' (Bevan 2006) you put into your work. This is the degree to which you are personally committed to helping your organisation by putting in more effort than is actually required to do your job. You are willing to do more, and you actually want to. What affects this is your interest, motivation, dedication, commitment and loyalty to your patients/clients and employer(s).

Interest 4: asking serious questions

This interest was essentially about how we get to do things differently and about, fundamentally, doing different things. It celebrated the art of question posing, frame-shifting, individual and collective critical and creative capabilities and moral courage. Although I talk about this in more detail later, I'll say this now: moral courage is about responding positively to a 'serious question' and about embracing the challenges of taking action. This interest also addresses the 'political' dimension that appears to be missing in Schön's work. By 'political', I mean the processes and patterns of power and behaviours that regulate who gets and does what, where, when and how. In *Developing the Reflective Healthcare Team* (Ghaye 2005), I set out eight of the qualities that characterise a serious question. Different questions may exhibit some or all of each of these eight qualities. A serious question is:

- *Your question:* You have some personal interest and professional stake in asking it.
- *Value-laden:* It expresses your value position in relation to the content of the question.
- *Ethically situated:* It is about what's best to do, for whom and why, with regard to a particular aspect of your work.
- *Critical:* The question is a challenging one in that it embraces a language of critique, critiquing the status quo, habit and taken-for-grantedness, imposition, inequality, oppressive work patterns, and so on.
- *Power-infused:* A serious question can help individuals and teams look again at how they relate to each other. They can help staff to free themselves from themselves.
- *Creative:* It can help change customary ways of thinking and doing things. Serious questions with this quality embrace a language of possibility.
- *One to be asked:* The seriousness of such questions inspires us to frame them in the most intelligible way possible and seek out opportunities to ask them. Seriousness has to be not only communicated but also heard.
- *Deserving of a response:* The seriousness conveyed in the question's message and medium (what is said and how) encourages those to whom it is directed to respond. It cannot be ignored. Others feel obliged to respond.

Serious questions asked by Plsek **et al.**

In their work for the UK's NHS Modernising Agency, Plsek *et al.* (2004) ask the following questions. How far would you regard them as embracing some of the above eight qualities of 'seriousness'?

- *Relationships:* Do the interactions among the various parts of the system generate energy and innovative ideas for change, or do they drain the organisation?
- *Decision-making:* Are decisions about change made rapidly and by the people with the most knowledge of the issue, or is change bogged down in a treacle of hierarchy and position-authority?
- *Power:* Do individuals and groups acquire and exercise power in positive, constructive ways toward a collective purpose, or is power coveted and used mainly for self-interest and self-preservation?
- *Conflict:* Are conflicts and differences of opinion embraced as opportunities to discover new ways of working, or are these seen as negative and destructive?

Moving on and building a new positive core

This book contains a development of these 'four interests'. I have re-framed and further clarified them in order to prepare the way for a consideration of how we might scale up these 'interests' so that reflective practices have the potential to become an organisation-wide work habit. Henceforth, 'interests' are more accurately and understandably called 'intentions'. So, what are they and what does each intention mean? These are set out in Table 1.8. It is important to remember that these intentions are not mutually exclusive. Learning replaces the word 'practice'. The four principle intentions form the basis of the positive core of reflective learning.

Table 1.9 co-relates these intentions with the scale of reflective learning. Data for the table have been drawn from 562 papers submitted for review (2000–06) to the international peer-reviewed journal *Reflective Practice*. Scale ranges from individualistic through to systemic. During the first six years of the journal's life, the editorial board has received four times as many papers documenting work at the scale of the individual than at the scale of the group/team or the whole organisation.

Reflective learning at the scale of the individual

There are, of course, many reasons for working at the scale of the individual, for example the historical roots and pervasiveness of reflection as an individualistic pursuit as captured in the label the 'reflective practitioner'. Another reason is associated with the personal, professional and practical challenges of scaling up reflection to involve groups of staff in

Table 1.8 Positive core of reflective learning.

Principle intentions (these are not mutually exclusive)	Description
1. To appreciate	This is inspired by Schön (1983) and Dewey's (1933) work on the reflective practitioner and more recently by work on appreciative enquiry (Cooperrider & Whitney 2005) and appreciative intelligence (Thatchenkery & Metzker 2006). It is an intention to appreciate and understand one's own and others' gifts, talents, limitations, self-worth, identity, role, responsibilities and accountability. It is an intention to develop a deeper understanding of one's own learning agenda, sense of self, self-knowledge, self-efficacy and purpose. The intention is to deepen appreciations.
2. To re-frame	The intention is to use the practices of reflection to generate, manage and utilise knowledge, re-frame it and then record this in some way. This is essentially done through reflective accounts and conversations of one kind or another, for example through narratives, diaries, logs, portfolios, essays, problem-based learning assignments and case-based scenarios. The intention is to document learning about what works, about problems, about how to improve practice, who to involve and why. It is associated with seeing with fresh eyes. This intention weaves together new or different ways of thinking, talking and working. Doing this involves learning to 'let go' and to 'welcome in'.
3. To build collective wisdom	This intention can be influenced positively by intentions 1 and 2. It harnesses individual expertise and connects 'islands of innovation', bringing both together into a new wholeness of collective wisdom. Criticality and creativity are required along with a preparedness to question conviction-laden practices and policies. Building collective wisdom requires emotional literacy, political acuity and ethical courage.
4. To achieve and move forward	The intention here is to do or achieve something with this collective wisdom, bearing in mind the issues raised earlier about reflection and action. It involves putting to good use new or different ways envisioned and documented. This intention is often associated with award-bearing assessments, fitness-to-practise, revalidation and meeting clinical standards. Achieving implies moving forward. This may be described and judged as incremental or as a step-change.

Table 1.9 Linking intentions with the potential scale of reflective learning.

Principle intentions of the practices of reflection	Scale of reflective learning		
	Individual (e.g. self)	Team (e.g. work-group/team, community)	Organisation (e.g. acute, primary care trust, general practice surgery)
1. To appreciate			
2. To re-frame			
3. To build collective wisdom			
4. To achieve and move forward			

more open, discursive and, therefore, more public reflections on practice. Allied to this are a range of concerns about privacy vis-à-vis, the right to know, litigation and whistle-blowing, among others, which may be of more concern with reflection at a greater scale. Another would be that we may need more courage, insight and support in working together in communities of reflective practitioners. We may need more courage and clarity of purpose to enable us to draw upon reflective practices on a larger, albeit usually more complex, scale. We do not have to see this as a burden on reflection or on ourselves. Interestingly, between 2004 and 2006, there has been a noticeable increase in papers submitted in healthcare that have begun to scale up the practices of reflection to the level of the workgroup or team. This mirrors the growth of more team-based work, the development of team cultures and the resultant flatter organisational structures in the UK NHS.

Tables 1.10 to 1.12 begin to illuminate the links between principle intentions and scale. I have used abstracts drawn from recently published papers in *Reflective Practice* to show this. No paper fits neatly into one 'box'. I have positioned them according to the main thrust or focus of the work.

To date, the journal has received very few publishable papers in healthcare where the practices of reflection are being used across the whole, or within noticeable parts, of the organisation. This does not mean it is not happening. But if it is, where are the accounts of it happening? Are we looking in the wrong place? Or are accounts simply not being written up and placed in the public domain?

Table 1.10 Illuminations of the four principle intentions of reflective learning at the scale of the INDIVIDUAL.

Principle intentions of reflective learning	Scale of reflective learning: THE INDIVIDUAL
1. To appreciate	Lindsay (2006) Reflecting on and reconstructing her experience from the late 1980s as a director of nursing who implemented family-centred care in a hospital, the author discerns narrative resonances with her contemporary life as a nurse-teacher. Through telling multiple versions of that story, intersecting with ongoing life events in the 1990s, she shows how identity is constructed and pulls forward into her teaching–learning practices in the new millennium. Telling the stories of family-centred care is, for the author, a way to uncover her assumptions that become fixed plotlines underpinning her actions. Her secret and cover stories emerge from daily life in social situations and show personal–professional connections. This paper explores the questions 'How does it matter to the nurse-teacher identity to reflect on and reconstruct life experience?' and 'How is this significant for shaping baccalaureate nursing curriculum?'
2. To re-frame	Wright (2005) This study examines master's students' perceptions of keeping a reflective journal (referred to here as a 'learning log') in initial and continuing psychotherapeutic training. In line with education, medical and management training, among others, the use of a learning log has become an established part of initial and continuing professional development in counselling and psychotherapy. If expressive and reflective, writing in this context is considered to be a significant part of the development of reflective practitioners in counselling. Additionally, psychotherapy questions arise about its facilitation and assessment in relation to student perceptions.

3. To build collective wisdom	Heron (2005) This article explores the connection between reflection and a critical approach to social work practice. By critical social work practice is meant a refusal of/opposition to the interlocking relations of power that pervade social worker encounters with clients. Frequent mention is made in current social work literature of the importance of workers recognising their social location in challenging racial, class, gender, heterosexual and ableist structures of domination. Reflection on the privileges associated with social location is considered the cornerstone of such an anti-oppressive practice, and Kondradt's (1999) article on critical self-reflectivity provides an important theoretical contribution to, and articulation of, what this would actually look like. However, drawing on Foucault's recognition of the power–knowledge axis, and his conceptualisation of power's capillary form, the author argues that the possibility of resisting the reproduction of dominant power relations rests on an analysis of one's subjectivity and subject positions.
4. To achieve and move forward	Gully (2004) The author demonstrates how reflective writing as critical reflection can provide added insight to our practice when working with sexually abusive adolescents, and in conjunction with other forms of reflection enables us to learn and change, becoming more effective in what we do.

Table 1.11 Intentions at the scale of the TEAM.

Principle intentions of reflective learning	Scale of reflective learning: THE TEAM
1. To appreciate	Krmpotić; Schwind (2003) 'Every experience should do something to prepare a person for later experiences of a deeper and more expansive quality' (Dewey 1938, p. 47). In order to learn from our experiences we need to reflect upon and seek meaning within them. A serious personal illness is one such experience that warrants closer scrutiny. The focus here is on three nurse-teachers, myself and two co-participants, who have personally experienced a serious illness. Through stories, journals, drawings, conversations and emerging metaphors, my co-participants and I dig progressively deeper with the intent to find any meaning our illnesses may have in our personal and professional lives. As this is a work in progress, only the preliminary process and outcomes are outlined.
2. To re-frame	McLean & Whalley (2004) This paper explores the evolution of a supervisory relationship over a period of two years. This relationship centred on a non-hierarchical way of sharing ideas and views, with the roles of 'supervisee' and 'supervisor' alternating in a flexible way of working, which may be described as 'co-supervision'. Through continued conversations between the authors and with colleagues, work together in co-supervision moved towards the development of a four-stage approach to co-supervision, which incorporated a reflective silence and a reflective conversation into the co-supervisory meetings. Engagement in co-supervision also modified ideas around evaluation methodology; the authors noticed a gradual shift from initial thoughts around a content analysis of the words and themes of co-supervision to a consideration of personal experiences in a more reflective way, hence this account. Finally, and importantly, the authors found that this evolving process had a positive effect upon psychotherapeutic relationships with mental health service users. In summary, this paper outlines the 'story' of one co-supervision relationship and reflects the narrative approach that underpins this work.

3. To build collective wisdom	**Nelson & Gould (2005)** This article presents the results of a series of conversations between two social scientists who undertake research with socially marginalised women with breast cancer. The paper highlights emergent themes from these discussions, including reflections about power relations and privilege, as well as facets of identity that come into play in the work, including race, class, gender, cultural capital and personal life histories. They reflect on the responsibilities within their work, which has social change as its end goal. The article considers several key questions, including 'How do our subjectivities and identities influence the choices we have made in our work?', 'How do these identities and their meanings change over time, and how is this incorporated in the work?' and 'How does reflection on these issues inform, challenge and change our research and its outcomes?' Finally, they reflect on how debriefing with one another has served as a reminder that factors influencing research processes and outcomes are larger and more intimately interwoven than is often apparent.
4. To achieve and move forward	**Sparrow & Heel (2006)** Team learning is a process through which teams engage in collective reflection and exploration of their perceptions. The practice, however, raises additional social psychological considerations of impression management and trust, together with a different dynamic within group interaction. Dialogue theory provides some principles concerning a means to *contain* potentially overwhelming aspects of reflection and disclosure necessary to promote reflection, openness and learning. This study reports an attempt by an individual within his own workplace (a UK specialist acute children's hospital) to facilitate the use of an effective process among 15 participants to develop their team learning practices over a period of more than two years. The development process highlighted four key concepts within team learning development: (i) knowledge sharing, (ii) work culture and environment, (iii) action and (iv) personal competence. A number of cycles and phases within each of these facets become apparent.

Table 1.12 Intentions at the scale of the ORGANISATION.

Principle intentions of reflective learning	Scale of reflective learning: **THE ORGANISATION**
1. To appreciate	Melander-Wikman *et al.* (2006) This is a reflective account of aspects of our collective concern about developing and sustaining ways that might enable elderly people to feel more empowered to exercise their right of self-determination. This work has been undertaken in the context of home healthcare in northern Sweden. In this paper we put three espoused values under pressure from client, professional (homecare staff) and research perspectives. We also explore three aspects of the landscape of homecare. They are the notions of client participation, empowerment and ICT. The live data for this paper are drawn from two days of workshop activities with 35 homecare staff working in the municipality of Luleå, Sweden. The workshop was one outcome of the e-Home Health Care @ North Calotte (eHHC) Project of 2003–05. We conclude with some collective reflections about (i) the *practice* of participation (dialogue) and an *intention* of it (empowerment) in the context of clients accelerating service change; (ii) how to re-frame traditional views of the relationships between research and practice and, as a consequence, open up new possibilities for understanding how elderly people's lived experiences can be a positive force for service improvement; and (iii) the use of storyboards as an appreciative approach to enable frontline staff to reflect on their work, share and learn together.
2. To re-frame	No adequate examples yet received

3. To build
collective wisdom

Sparrow et al. (2005)
An increasing number of academic and professional development programmes engender reflective practice. There is little doubt that participants leave such programmes equipped and keen to utilise reflective practice in their own workplace practices. There is evidence to suggest, however, that the workplace itself may conspire to limit the extent to which reflection is practised. Reflecting at a meta-level upon why and how reflective practice is inhibited may be valuable in helping reflective practitioners secure more widespread reflection at work. This paper reports a methodology for an exploration of the workplace features of an NHS manager's job that determined the 'reflective space' in his work sphere. The study involved a provisional classification of work events where reflection was notably high or low and the subsequent use of the repertory grid procedure to elicit the personal constructs of this notion of reflective space. A principal components analysis and factor analysis of the repertory grid data indicated five major characteristics of the reflective practitioner's workplace that can inhibit or facilitate reflective practice. These were the degrees of prescriptiveness: engagement; role-based, demarcated and political features; threat; and task versus process orientation. A discussion of the implications of these findings is made.

4. To achieve and
move forward

No adequate examples yet received

References

Ackoff, R. (1979) The future of operational research is past. *Journal of the Operational Research Society* **30**, 93–104.

Albanese, M.A. (2006) Crafting the reflective lifelong learner: why, what and how. *Medical Education* **40**(4), 288–90.

Allan, J., Pease, B. & Briskman, L. (eds) (2003) *Critical Social Work: An Introduction to Theories and Practices*. Allen & Unwin, Crows Nest, NSW, Australia.

Amos, D. (2006) Don't be bitten by the bench. *Health Service Journal*, 27 July, 32.

Argyris, C. & Schön, D. (1976) *Theory in Practice: Increasing Professional Effectiveness*. Jossey-Bass, San Francisco, CA.

Barnett, R. (1997) *Higher Education: A Critical Business*. Open University Press, Buckingham.

Berwick, D.M. (2004) Lessons from developing nations on improving health care. *British Medical Journal* **328**, 1124–9.

Bevan, H. (2006) Helen Bevan on motivation and productivity. *Health Service Journal*, 30 March, 23.

Bleakley, A. (2002) Pre-registration house officers and ward-based learning: a 'new apprenticeship' model. *Medical Education* **36**(1), 9–15.

Boyd, E. & Fales, A. (1983) Reflective learning: key to learning experience. *Journal of Humanistic Psychology* **23**(2), 99–117.

Brookfield, S. (1990) Using critical incidents to explore learners' assumptions. In *Fostering Critical Reflection in Adulthood* (ed. J. Mezirow). Jossey-Bass, San Francisco, CA.

Brookfield, S. (1995a) *Becoming a Critically Reflective Teacher*. Jossey-Bass, San Francisco, CA.

Brookfield, S. (1995b) *Developing Critical Thinkers: Challenging Adults to Explore Alternative Ways of Thinking and Acting*. Open University Press, Buckingham.

Brookfield, S. (2000a) The concept of critically reflective practice. In *Handbook of Adult and Continuing Education* (eds A.L. Wilson & E.R. Hayes). Jossey-Bass, San Francisco, CA.

Brookfield, S. (2000b) Transformative learning as ideology critique. In *Learning as Transformation: Critical Perspectives on a Theory in Progress* (ed. J. Mezirow). Jossey-Bass, San Francisco, CA.

Bulman, C. (2004) *Reflective Practice in Nursing: The Growth of the Professional Practitioner*. Blackwell Publishing, Oxford.

Carr, W. & Kemmis, S. (1986) *Becoming Critical: Education, Knowledge and Action Research*. Falmer Press, Lewes.

Clift, E (ed.) (2005) *Women, Philanthropy and Social Change: Visions for a Just Society*. University Press of New England, Hanover, NH.

Cooperrider, D. & Whitney, D. (2005) *Appreciative Inquiry: A Positive Revolution in Change*. Berrett-Koehler, San Francisco, CA.

Cossentino, J. (2002) Importing artistry: further lessons from the design studio. *Reflective Practice* **3**(1), 39–52.

Day, C. (1999) Researching teaching through reflective practice. In *Researching Teaching: Methodologies and Practices for Understanding Pedagogy* (ed. J. Loughran). Falmer Press, London.

Dewey, J. (1916) *Democracy and Education*. The Free Press, New York.

Dewey, J. (1933) *How We Think: A Restatement of the Relation of Reflective Thinking to the Educative Process*. Henrey Regney, Chicago, IL.

Dewey, J. (1938) (reprinted 1963). *Experience and Education*. Macmillan, New York.

Dewey, J. (1973) *The Philosophy of John Dewey* (ed. J. McDermott). Putnam Sons, New York.

Dominelli, L (2002) *Feminist Social Work Theory and Practice*. Palgrave, Basingstroke.

Eisner, E.W. (1985) *The Art of Educational Evaluation: A Personal View*. Falmer Press, London.

Eraut, M. (1995) Schön shock: a case for refraining reflection-in-action? *Teachers and Teaching: Theory and Practice* **1**(1), 9–22.

Eraut, M., Steadman, S., Furner, J., *et al.* (2004) Early career learning at work: the LiNEA Project. Presented at the TLRP Conference, Cardiff, 22–24 November 2004.

Fay, B. (1987) *Critical Social Science*. Cornell University Press, Ithaca, NY.

Fish, D. & de Cossart, L. (2006) Thinking outside the (tick) box: rescuing professionalism and professional judgement. *Medical Education* **40**(5), 403–4.

Fook, J. (1993) *Radical Casework*. Allen & Unwin, St Leonards.

Fook, J. (1996) (ed.) *The Reflective Researcher: Social Workers' Theories of Practice Research*. Allen & Unwin, Sydney.

Fook, J. (2002) *Critical Social Work*. Sage, London.

Freire, P. (1972) *Pedagogy of the Oppressed*. Sheed and Ward, London.

Freire, P. (1974) *Education for Critical Consciousness*. Sheed and Ward, London.

Freire, P. (1994) *Pedagogy of Hope*. Continuum, New York.

Freire, P. (1998) *Pedagogy of the Heart*. Continuum, New York.

Freshwater, D. (ed.) (2002) *Therapeutic Nursing*. Sage, London.

Ghaye, T. (2005) *Developing the Reflective Healthcare Team*. Blackwell Publishing, Oxford.

Ghaye, T. & Lillyman, S. (2000) *Reflection: Principles and Practice for Healthcare Professionals*. Mark Allen, Dinton, UK.

Ghaye, T. & Lillyman, S. (2006a) *Learning Journals and Critical Incidents: Reflective Practice for Healthcare Professionals*, 2nd edn. Mark Allen, Dinton, UK.

Ghaye, T. & Lillyman, S. (2006b) *Reflection and Writing a Reflective Account*. CD-ROM. IRP-UK Publications, Gloucester.

Gibbs, G. (1988) *Learning by Doing: A Guide to Teaching and Learning Methods*. Further Education Unit, Oxford Brookes University, Oxford.

Gilbert, D. (2006) *In Pursuit of Happiness*. HarperCollins, London.

Gleick, J. (1991) *Chaos*. Sphere Books, London.

Gully, T. (2004) Reflective writing as critical reflection in work with sexually abusive adolescents. *Reflective Practice* **5**(3), 313–26.

Habermas, J. (1974) *Theory and Practice* (trans. J. Vientall). Heinemann, London.

Hart, G. & Rotem, A. (1995) The clinical learning environment: nurses perceptions of professional development in clinical settings. *Nurse Education Today* **15**, 3–10.

Heron, B. (2005) Self reflection in critical social work practice: subjectivity and the possibilities of resistance. *Reflective Practice* **6**(3), 341–51.

Hick, S., Fook, J. & Pozzuto, R. (eds) (2005) *Social Work: A Critical Turn*. Thompson, Toronto.

Higgs, J. & Andresen, L. (2001) The knower, the knowing and the known: threads in the woven tapestry of knowledge. In *Practice Knowledge and Expertise in the Health Professions* (eds J. Higgs and A. Titchen). Butterworth-Heinemann, Oxford.

Ife, J. (1997) *Rethinking Social Work: Towards Critical Practice*. Longman, Melbourne.

Jasper, M. (2007) *Vital Notes for Nurses: Professional Development, Reflection and Decision-Making*. Blackwell Publishing, Oxford.

Johns, C. (2001) Reflective Practice: revealing the [he]art of caring. *International Journal of Nursing Practice* **7**(4), 237–45.

Johns, C. (2002) *Guided Reflection: Advancing Practice*. Blackwell Science, Oxford.

Johns, C. (2004) *Becoming a Reflective Practitioner*. Blackwell Publishing, Oxford.

Johns, C. (2006) *Engaging Reflection in Practice*. Blackwell Publishing, Oxford.

Johns, C. & Freshwater, D. (eds) (1998) *Transforming Nursing Through Reflective Practice*. Blackwell Publishing, Oxford.

Jones, M. (2003) Reflective practice and learning: an education program for school nurses. Unpublished paper. Deakin University, Geelong, Australia.

King, P. & Kitchener, K. (1994) *Developing Reflective Judgement*. Jossey-Bass, San Francisco, CA.

Kolb, D.A. and Fry, R. (1975) Toward an applied theory of experiential learning. In *Theories of Group Process* (ed. C. Cooper). John Wiley & Sons, London.

Kondradt, M.E. (1999) Who is the 'self' in self-aware: professional self-awareness from a critical theory perspective. *Social Service Review* **73**, 451–77.

Kraft, N.P. (1997) A critical analysis of the role change agents in facilitating change. Unpublished doctoral dissertation. University of Wisconsin, Madison, WI.

Kraft, N.P. (2002) Teacher research as a way to engage in critical reflection: a case study. *Reflective Practice* **3**(2), 175–89.

Krmpotić Schwind, J. (2003) Reflective process in the study of illness stories as experienced by three nurse teachers. *Reflective Practice* **4**(1), 19–32.

Larrivee, B. (2000) Transforming teaching practice: becoming the critically reflective teacher. *Reflective Practice* **1**(3), 285–307.

Leonard, P. (1997) *Postmodern Welfare: Reconstructing the Emancipatory Project*. Sage, London.

Lindsay, G. (2006) Constructing a nursing identity: reflecting on and reconstructing experience. *Reflective Practice* **7**(1), 59–72.

Loughran, J. (2006) A response to 'Reflecting on the self'. *Reflective Practice* **7**(1), 43–53.

Luke, A. (2004) Two takes on the critical. In *Critical Pedagogies and Language Learning* (eds B. Norton & K. Toohey). Cambridge University Press, Cambridge.

Maister, D., Galford, R.M. & Green, C.H. (2002) *The Trusted Advisor*. Simon & Schuster, London.

Mamede, S. & Schmidt, H.G. (2004) The structure of reflective practice in medicine. *Medical Education* **38**(12), 1302–8.

Marchant, H. & Wearing, B. (eds) (1986) *Gender Reclaimed: Women in Social Work*. Hale & Iremonger, Sydney.

McCormack, B. (2001) 'The dangers of a missing chapter': a journey of discovery through reflective practice. *Reflective Practice* **2**(2), 209–19.

McLean, B. & Whalley, J. (2004) No real tale has a beginning or an end . . . exploring the relationship between co-supervision, reflective dialogue and psychotherapeutic work with mental health service users. *Reflective Practice* **5**(2), 225–38.

Melander-Wikman, A., Jansson, M. & Ghaye, T. (2006) Reflections on an appreciative approach to empowering elderly people, in home healthcare. *Reflective Practice* **7**(4), 423–44.

Mezirow, J. (1978) Perspective transformation. *Adult Education* **28**, 100–110.

Mezirow, J. (1981) A critical theory of adult learning and education. *Adult Education* **32**(1), 3–24.

Mezirow, J. (1990) *Fostering Critical Reflection in Adulthood: A Guide to Transformative and Emancipatory Learning*. Jossey-Bass, San Francisco, CA.

Moon, J. (2004) *A Handbook of Reflective and Experiential Learning: Theory and Practice*. RoutledgeFalmer, London.

Moreau, M. (1979) A structural approach to social work practice. *Canadian Journal of Social Work Education* **5**(1), 78–93.

Morley, C. (2007) Cross-disciplinary critical reflection: issues and dilemmas. *Reflective Practice* **8**(1), 61–74.

Mullaly, B. (1993) *Structural Social Work: Ideology, Theory and Practice*. McClelland & Stewart, Toronto.

Mullaly, B. (2002) *Challenging Oppression: A Critical Social Work Approach*. Oxford University Press, Don Mills, Ontario.

Nelson, J. & Gould, J. (2005) Hidden in the mirror: a reflective conversation about research with marginalized communities. *Reflective Practice* **6**(3), 327–39.

O'Hanlon, C. (1994) Reflection and action in research: is there a moral responsibility to act? *Educational Action Research* **2**(2), 281–9.

Parker, S. (1997) *Reflective Teaching in the Postmodern World*. Open University Press, Buckingham.

Pease, B. & Fook, J. (eds) (1999) *Transforming Social Work Practice: Postmodern Critical Perspectives*. Allen & Unwin, St Leonards.

Plsek, P., Bibby, J. & Garrett, S. (2004) *Mapping Behavioural Patterns, Summary Booklet*. NHS Modernisation Agency, London.

Pollard, A. (2002) *Reflective Teaching: Effective and Evidence-Informed Professional Practice*. Continuum, London.

Pollard, A. (2005) *Reflective Teaching: Evidence Informed Professional Practice*, 2nd edn. Continuum, London.

Reynolds, M. & Vince, R. (eds) (2004) *Organizing Reflection*. Ashgate Publishing, Aldershot.

Rider, E.A. & Brashers, V. (2006) Team-based learning: a strategy for interprofessional collaboration. *Medical Education* **40**(5), 486–7.

Rolfe, G., Freshwater, D. & Jasper, M. (2001) *Critical Reflection for Nursing and the Helping Professions: A User's Guide*. Palgrave, Basingstoke.

Schön, D. (1983) *The Reflective Practitioner: How Professionals Think in Action*. Basic Books, New York.

Schön, D. (1987) *Educating the Reflective Practitioner: Towards a New Design for Teaching and Learning in the Professions*. Jossey-Bass, San Francisco, CA.

Schön, D. (ed.) (1991) *The Reflective Turn*. Teachers College Press, New York.

Senge, P., Scharmer, C., Jaworski. J. & Flowers, B. (2005) *Presence: An Exploration of Profound Change in People, Organisations, And Society*. Doubleday, New York.

Sinclair-Penwarden, A. (2006) Listen up: we should not be made to disclose our personal feelings in reflection assignments. *Nursing Times* **102**(37), 12.

Smyth, J. (1991) *Teachers as Collaborative Learners*. Open University Press, Milton Keynes.

Sobral, D. (2000) An appraisal of medical students' reflection-in-learning. *Medical Education* **34**(3), 182–7.

Sparrow, J. & Heel, D. (2006) Fostering team learning development. *Reflective Practice* **7**(2), 151–62.

Sparrow, J., Ashford, R. & Heel, D. (2005) A methodology to identify workplace features that can facilitate or impede reflective practice: a National Health Service UK study. *Reflective Practice* **6**(2), 189–97.

Stewart, I. (1995) *Nature's Numbers: Discovering Order and Pattern in the Universe*. Weidenfeld & Nicholson, London.

Stewart, I. & Golubitsky, M. (1992) *Complexity: The Emerging Science at the Edge of Order and Chaos*. Simon & Schuster, New York.

Stuart, C.C. (2001) The reflective journeys of a midwifery tutor and her students. *Reflective Practice* **2**(2), 171–84.

Thatchenkery, T. & Metzker, C. (2006) *Appreciative Intelligence: Seeing the Mighty Oak in the Acorn*. Berrett-Koehler, San Francisco, CA.

Tripp, D. (1998) Critical incidents in action inquiry in ethnography. In *Being Reflexive and Critical in Educational and Social Research* (eds J. Smyth & G. Shacklock). Falmer Press, London.

Valkenburg, R. & Dorst, K. (1998) The reflective practice of design teams. *Design Studies* **19**(3), 249–71.

Van Den Bergh, N. & Cooper, L.B. (eds) (1986) *Feminist Visions for Social Work*. National Association of Social Workers, Silver Spring, MD.

van Manen, M. (1994). Pedagogy, virtue, and narrative identity in teaching. *Curriculum Inquiry* **4**(2), 135–70.

van Manen, M. (1995) On the epistemology of reflective practice. *Teachers and Teaching: Theory and Practice* **1**(1), 33–49.

van Manen, M. (1999) The practice of practice. In *Changing Schools, Changing Practices: Perspectives on Educational Reform and Teacher Professionalism* (ed. M. Lang). Garant, Luvain, Belgium.

Watson, J. (1999) *Postmodern Nursing and Beyond*. Churchill Livingstone, Edinburgh.

Whitehead, J. (2000) How do I improve my practice? Creating and legitimating an epistemology of practice. *Reflective Practice* **1**(1), 91–104.

Wright, J. (2005) 'A discussion with myself on paper': counselling and psychotherapy masters student perceptions of keeping a learning log. *Reflective Practice* **6**(4), 507–21.

Zebrack, J. & Fletcher, K.E. (2006) Competency pocket cards: an effective ambulatory assessment tool. *Medical Education* **40**(5), 480–81.

Zeichner, M. & Liston, D. (1996) *Reflective Teaching: An Introduction.* Lawrence Erlbaum, Mahwah, NJ.

Chapter 2

Action step 2: r-learning as an innovation

In this second action step over the 'rough ground', I frame the process of building a reflective healthcare organisation as a process of innovation. This action step contains two major ideas bundles:

Bundle 1 **Successful innovations**
This invites you to regard the scaling up of r-learning as a process of innovation. For some, this implies a *big change*, which is different from incremental change. In some healthcare organisations, such an audacious goal would be regarded as a large-scale transformation; in others, it would be considered a significant departure from current practice. Scaling up r-learning so that it becomes a collegial and useful organisation-wide work habit requires us to think differently. Framing the process as an innovation and actively learning from innovation theory is just that. The bundle explores the basic elements of the spread of any innovation, namely, the coverage and the uptake of it. Various conceptions of the process of adoption are presented, along with Rogers' important set of criteria for judging the success of such a process. The processes are illustrated from work in healthcare.

Bundle 2 **Scaling up**
This bundle defines scaling up as an activity of increasing access to, uptake of and impact on more and more people, over time, across a healthcare organisation, of r-learning. Scaling up means transforming reflection from an individualistic practice into a self-sustaining, collective learning process. The bundle contains two views of a scaling-up process: staged and non-linear.

To help you navigate your way through action step 2, these ideas are conveyed in a simple mind map (Fig. 2.1).

The fight against scurvy

For many centuries, scurvy was the main threat to the health of naval crews. When Vasco de Gama sailed around the Cape of Good Hope for the first time in 1497, 100 of his crew of 160 men died of scurvy. Nobody knew about vitamin C at that time, but some dietary factor was suspected. Captain James Lancaster proved it in 1601, when commanding a fleet of four ships on a voyage from England to India. On that voyage, the crew on one ship were given three teaspoons of

(Continued)

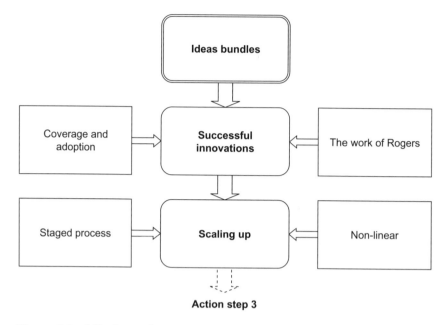

Figure 2.1   Mind map for action step 2: r-learning as an innovation.

lemon juice every day. At the halfway point on the trip, 110 (40 per cent) of 278 sailors on the other three ships had died of scurvy, but none died on the ship with the ration of lemon juice.

However, no one seemed to notice: despite Lancaster's evidence, practices in the British navy did not change. The study was repeated 146 years later, in 1747, by a British navy physician named James Lind. In a random trial of six treatments for scorbutic sailors on the HMS Salisbury, citrus again proved effective against scurvy. It took the British navy 48 more years to react by ordering that citrus fruits become a part of the diet on all navy ships. Scurvy in the British navy disappeared almost overnight. The British Board of Trade took 70 more years to adopt the innovation, ordering proper diets on merchant marine vessels in 1865. The total time elapsed from Lancaster's definitive study to universal British preventive policy on scurvy was 264 years (Berwick 2003, pp. 1969–70).

Coverage and uptake of innovations

In this chapter I work with the idea that scaling up r-learning so that it becomes an organisation-wide sustainable work habit can be regarded as a *process of innovation*. So what does the fight against scurvy tell us about the coverage and uptake of innovations? Let's clarify the language first. In a paper by Pokhrel (2006), the scaling up of health services has two facets.

The first is extending the availability of cost-effective interventions to a chosen population; this is about *coverage*. The second facet is concerned with increasing the level of demand for these services; this is about *uptake*. Pokhrel goes on to argue that improving the supply of interventions is a necessary condition in any scaling-up process. But understanding uptake of services is critical. Coverage and uptake are two basic ideas associated with the process of scaling up. In the context of this book, coverage is linked with *who* is participating in r-learning – in other words, which individuals and teams, in which parts of the organisation. Coverage is about how far it has *spread*. Basically, this has *within* and *between* aspects. The former is about more and more staff within the same area of work embracing r-learning, for example within a community drug and alcohol team or within a paediatric intensive care unit. It can also mean spread within a particular team of health visitors, Macmillan nurses or occupational therapists and so on. Between aspects refer to the spread of r-learning between stakeholder groups, clinical teams and directorates and across localities, for example between those involved in improving working lives, with equality and diversity, in planning and delivering integrated care pathways, risk management, hospital cleanliness, patient and public involvement, and so on. Essentially, spread needs to be thought of as bringing the quality benefits of r-learning to staff, across the organisation, equitably and lastingly. Spread is *not* synonymous with copying.

The rate of adoption

Uptake is about *how many* staff are engaging in r-learning. This is linked with the notion of an 'innovation' and to a process called the 'rate of adoption'. I suggest that building a reflective healthcare organisation requires us to frame r-learning as an innovation that needs to be communicated (or diffused) throughout all of an organisation's functioning parts over time and adopted among its staff. In a reflective healthcare organisation, r-learning is a visible and sustained process. It has been adopted across the organisation and is felt to be a necessary and valuable collective work habit. How well the principle intentions and benefits of r-learning are communicated to others, and the understandings staff have of it, will often determine its rate of adoption. Often there is a 'gap' between what we have and what we could have. Berwick (2003) asks a fundamental question around the issue of the gap between our knowledge of something (e.g. an innovation) and putting the knowledge to good use in practice:

> Why do clinical care systems not incorporate the findings of clinical science or copy 'best known' practices reliably, quickly and even gratefully into their daily work, simply as a matter of course?

(Berwick 2003, p. 1969)

Until recently, the potency of r-learning was often determined by the subjective evaluation or 'feel-good factor' of those using it. So its spread from one staff group to another often depended upon near-peers' feelings and thoughts rather than upon any clear, evidence-based connections between r-learning and service improvement. It was a kind of mindset characterised by 'If it worked for them, then it's likely to work for us' or 'If they liked it, then the chances are we'll like it too.' But things are changing. I'll come back to this point later.

Framing r-learning as an innovation

Understanding how we can scale up reflective learning so that it becomes an organisation-wide, sustainable work habit requires a deep appreciation of two things: the notion of an innovation and the process of adoption. In what sense, then, could r-learning be described as an innovation? Nutley *et al.* (2002) offer four ways of understanding the notion of an innovation. I illustrate them here and then align each one with r-learning.

- *Innovation as developmental:* This is about modifying or improving what is already in existence with regard to an existing group. Charters and Pellegrin (1972) call this 'reinvention' or 'adaptation'. Clinically it might be the use of a different drug for existing patients with chronic diseases such as gastric ulcers or depression. With r-learning, it might be to improve the process by modifying the way an existing (reflective) team uses its meeting time, for example by making such meetings more focused.
- *Innovation as expansionary:* This is expanding or spreading that which already exists. Clinically it might be the greater provision of contraceptive services to younger people in order to reduce teenage pregnancies, or the development of a trauma stabilisation unit for people with fractures, or the expansion of orthopaedic services to reduce waiting times for emergency orthopaedic patients. With regard to r-learning, it might be about more and/or different staff embracing the process as a good work habit.
- *Innovation as evolutionary:* This is where something new is provided to an existing group. Clinically this might be the use of the drug Herceptin® for women with early-stage breast cancer, or the provision of a new centre for liquid cytology to make the process of cervical smears more accurate. With r-learning, it might mean peer-group reflective conversations being introduced to replace private, one-to-one supervisor–supervisee conversations with an already known group of staff.
- *Innovation as total:* This is where something new is provided for a new group, for example the provision of a new Health on the Streets (HOTS) initiative to empower harder-to-reach groups to take more control over their own health, or the provision of a weekly inclusive 'Time For Me' service, where attendees can exercise, relax and learn about stress and weight management. With r-learning, it might mean

using case-based or scenario-based discussions to promote r-learning among a newly formed multidisciplinary team.

Innovation as a good thing

There are a number of assumptions embedded in what I've said about innovation. The first is the tendency to always, and often uncritically, see innovation as a 'good thing' (Osborne 1998). Is it always? Whatever your views, I suggest that we are compelled to ask the question 'What makes an innovation, such as r-learning, worth adopting?' (see below). From this stems another assumption: that we are always rational when we adopt a particular innovation. But this is not always so. It might be unwise to assume that we always make wise and efficient choices to adopt (or not). As mentioned earlier, we can be influenced by fads and fashion, what we think might be regarded as 'politically correct' behaviour, by the urge to 'join in' and jump on the current bandwagon, by misinformation and mis-interpretations of what the innovation is all about (Abrahamson 1991, 1996, O'Neill *et al.* 1998, Walshe & Rundall 2001, Westphal *et al.* 1997). Another embedded assumption is that innovations flow top-down, or from experts to novices, or from outside the organisation and in, and so on. Again, this is not always true. Further, it is assumed that the spread and take-up of an innovation, like r-learning as an organisation-wide pro-cess, can be described as a step-by-step, accumulative and linear process. Not so; it is much more complex than this. The scaling up of r-learning is affected by existing staff interactions, in the sense of existing patterns of behaviour, and also by the prevailing organisational mindscape, best sum-marised by its stated values. Where an expression of r-learning (in one guise or another) is espoused in an organisation's 'mission statement', 'aspirational vision', 'audacious goals' or simply 'our values', but is a poor fit with existing patterns of interaction, r-learning may well struggle to become a lived reality for staff. Where there is a goodness of fit between an organisation's espoused values and existing patterns of behaviour, con-ditions are usually more favourable for adoption.

The complexity of scaling up

Scaling up is a complex phenomenon. Berwick (2003, pp. 1969–75) elabor-ates upon this complexity by suggesting in healthcare that we:

- Find good innovations and know how best to do this.
- Find and support innovators as they are a key part in building a posi-tive future.
- Invest in early adopters, in curiosity rather than compliance.
- Make early-adopter activity observable so that the majority know what's going on.
- Trust and enable the customisation of innovations. Local adoption often means local adaptation.

- Create slack to enable change, as change requires extra energy.
- Lead by example. We should not expect others to change if we are not prepared to change ourselves.

There are two further things to add to this list. We:

- need to align innovations with organisational values;
- should be prepared for setbacks if an innovation, particularly if it is related to improving performance, is imposed upon existing patterns of behaviour.

As mentioned earlier, it is unwise to think that if we keep doing things the same way, we can expect improved or even different outcomes. I set out additional issues below.

What makes an innovation successful?

Let's take a big public health issue – that of obesity, and childhood obesity in particular. The latter has doubled in England over the past ten years, and one in four children is now obese. From 1995 to 2004, obesity in boys aged 11–15 years rose from 14 per cent to 24 per cent and in girls from 15 per cent to 26 per cent. The rate rose slightly in the age group of two to ten years (Weaver 2006). Some have described this as a health time-bomb. UK government ministers have said that more has to be done to hit the target to halt the rise in child obesity by 2010. In September 2006, the UK government set new nutritional standards for school lunches and other school food. These standards say that schools must:

- make high-quality meat, poultry or oily fish regularly available on their menus;
- serve pupils at least two portions of fruit and vegetables with every meal;
- limit deep-fried food to no more than two portions per week;
- remove fizzy drinks, crisps, chocolate and other confectioneries from school meals and vending machines.

The implementation of these standards can be regarded as an innovation in schools. The work of celebrity chef Jamie Oliver and his Feed Me Better campaign, which revealed the state of British school dinners, has also served to highlight healthy lunchtime eating as a genuine innovation. Here is a conversation among a small group of 13-year-old boys and girls attending an inner-city comprehensive school that I listened to. Within this conversation we can find many of the important characteristics of innovations that affect their coverage and take-up:

> **Alex:** *Farty beans, farty cabbage, farty sprouts. Fart, fart, fart! What are they trying to do? Stink the whole school out?*
>
> **Sam:** They can't force us to eat it. We'll just sit here and eat nothing – then see how they like it.

Chris: Yeah, they think our food's crap, so we'll show them this food's crap!
Sam: Why can't we just eat what we want? It's nothing to do with them.

Alex: Yeah, if I wanna fill my face with chips and chocolate who says I can't?
Ben: They think we're thick and we'll just say 'Oh, great. Fantastic! Healthy food! Give us more!'

Alex: Yeah, like ditch our perfectly OK menu, thank you, and we'll go 'Wow, we love this! Why didn't we think of eating rice every day with boiled greens and no chips?' Yeah, right.
Sam: My mum says she's gonna complain to Kenzie and tell him that he can't force us to eat this.

Chris: Yeah, but it's his school and he'll just say that he can do what he likes.
Sam: But he can't.

Alex: He can!
Sam: No, he can't! He's got to get the parents to agree or he can't afford it. I saw it on Jamie Oliver's TV programme.

Chris: Jamie Oliver? He should be banned from every school in the country!
Ben: Kenzie's only trying this food for a term.

Alex: So if we don't eat it, he'll have to bring back the old menu?
Ben: Get real. He keeps telling us we'll get fat if we eat 'junk' food.

Chris: Yeah, and get diabetes and have heart attacks. Like I'm bovvered!
Sam: He should prove it. If he wants to ban Coke and crisps he can prove they'll kill me first.

Alex: And then we'll bury you in a coffin full of Walkers and say 'Told you so! Smoky bacon, off you go!'
[laughter]
Ben: Kenzie should have warned us that he was changing the menu.

Chris: He chickened out! Get it? Chickened out!
[jeering]
Sam: Yeah, we might have started a junk-food revolution!

Ben: He should just have changed bits of it.
Alex: What's the point? I'm not fat and I haven't got diabetes!

Ben: Sam's fat!
Sam: Piss off!

Chris: Yeah, well you eat six packets of crisps a day and drink loads of Coke.
Sam: And you stuff your face with kebabs and chips. Like, who's really fat, Mr Blobby?

Ben: Miss 'thunder thighs' Thornton!
Alex: Yeah, Kenzie should make all the teachers eat this crap too.

Chris: And if Thornton loses weight, we'll all do it!
Ben: Dare you to ask Kenzie that one!

Chris: Deal! And if I win, you owe me a mega-sized kebab and an extra-large portion of chips!
Ben: Done!
[laughter as the friends get up from the table, pushing their plates away]

Important innovation-related questions

At least five important innovation-related questions arise from the conversation among these teenage pupils. They are:

- Can the healthy-eating campaign (the innovation) be perceived as an improvement?
- How far do the children involved have to change their existing eating habits?
- How difficult is it for children to understand why healthy eating matters?
- Have schools introduced the changes in the most appropriate way?
- What are the observable benefits to children?

Let's relate these questions more generally to healthcare innovations and to r-learning, as an innovation, in particular. Entire organisations in healthcare are devoted to promoting innovations, selling the latest drug, imaging system, medical device or software package. Additionally, we tend to keep an eye out for things such as the latest and best drugs, surgery and diagnostic strategy. Thus, the pace at which new ideas and technologies spread through various healthcare systems is of great interest as it affects costs, clinical outcomes and user satisfaction. In a time like this, of rapid healthcare reform, I often have discussions with staff about the difference between a change and an improvement. How would we know? All improvement is a change, but not all change can be regarded as an improvement. Additionally, how would we know that an innovation was an improvement? It may indeed herald changes, but this is not the same as saying that the innovation was 'right' for the organisation, its staff and service users, at this point in time. This begs the question 'What makes an innovation successful?' Sanson-Fisher (2004) reviews the earlier work of Rogers (1983) and sets out a number of critical characteristics that help us with this question. These are not requirements for a successful innovation; neither do they guarantee success. But their absence greatly effects coverage and up-take. The characteristics are:

- *Relative advantage:* Is the innovation (e.g. r-learning) better than what is currently in place? Is adopting it better than holding on to the status quo? How far will staff perceive r-learning as better than already existing processes, within the healthcare organisation, that support learning and development? If there is no relative advantage, r-learning will not spread quickly, if it spreads at all.
- *Compatibility:* This is tricky. On the one hand we could argue that the more compatible an innovation is with patterns of behaviour that already exist, the greater the prospects for its adoption and diffusion. But it may be that the innovation is indeed regarded as such and valued because changes in behaviour (patterns of interaction) are exactly

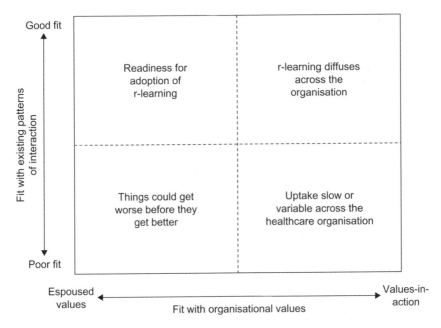

Figure 2.2 Framework for thinking about scaling up r-learning.

what it is intended to bring about. The central consideration is around the notion of 'fit' (Fig. 2.2), for example how far r-learning fits with people's past experiences (of, say, one-to-one clinical supervision), with present and future needs (of, say, better multidisciplinary team-work and learning). For me, the key question is 'How far does the adoption and diffusion of r-learning require a change in the organisation's existing values?' If staff feel they have to become very different people, engaging with others differently, conversing more openly, more optimistically, and so on, while working in a culture of disappointment and cynicism, then it is possible that r-learning (as an innovation) might meet with some resistance.

- *Complexity:* The most important question here is 'How difficult is it for staff to understand and use r-learning?' I was taught a tough lesson during a visit to New York when I had a conversation about 'r-learning' with the director of communications for Ogilvy & Mather, one of the world's largest international advertising, marketing and public relations agencies. I was invited to make a 30-second 'pitch' to convey the essence of it. I went over by 10 seconds; this was not well received. Did the audience of senior directors get it first time around? No, not everyone. I learned that it is relatively easy to make something sound complicated but hugely skilful to make complexity simple. The more complex r-learning is perceived to be, the greater the chance of slower adoption.
- *Trialability:* In times of financial stringency particularly, those who might invest in r-learning will wish to know what the return on their

investment will be. The investment may be in terms of time, energy, commitment, money, good will, and so on. It is important that staff are given an opportunity to try things out. Why should any organisation have to commit to r-learning all at once? If staff feel they do have to commit, then they are likely to be far more cautious about adopting it. The free samples that pharmaceutical companies distribute to healthcare professionals are an obvious example of using trialability to promote adoption. But what about r-learning? Trials might consist of one- or two-hour awareness-raising and taster sessions. They might involve a small group of key players understanding the principles and processes underpinning r-learning and how r-learning might add value to existing workstreams to which the organisation is already committed. Trials might be about 'having a go' with some reflective tools and techniques. They might involve committing to a taster session, followed by a cooling-off period (a time for in-house discussions about feasibility, applicability and benefit), which is followed later with a conversation about adoption (or not).

- *Observability:* One of the long-running debates within the field of learning through reflection and its practices has been about the difference it makes, to whom, in what way and when – in other words, with any kind of evidence that it makes an observable difference. The more obvious the evidence of improvement, the better the observable outcome, the more chance r-learning will be adopted by others.

Table 2.1 is a brief literature review of the various dimensions of an answer to the question 'What makes a successful innovation?' In this table I have reviewed the 'change knowledge' (Fullan 2005) from some of the leading research papers recording the experience of innovation processes in the private sector. It is a source of useful learning.

Reflecting on patient safety

A Department of Health report (2000) called 'An organisation with a memory' identified that the key barriers to reducing the number of patient safety incidents were an organisational culture that inhibited reporting and the lack of a cohesive national system for identifying and sharing lessons learnt. This report was an important milestone in the NHS's patient safety agenda and marked the drive to improve reporting and learning. As a consequence of this, the National Patient Safety Agency (NPSA) in the UK was launched in August 2001. This occurred in a broad context of concerns that the NHS had limited information about the extent and impact of clinical and non-clinical incidents and that NHS trusts needed to learn from these incidents and share good practice more effectively. The major contribution to care of the NPSA has been to develop national solutions that prevent incidents that affect

Table 2.1 What makes a successful innovation?

Innovation attributes	Adopter characteristics	Environmental/ context characteristics	Promoter characteristics	Communication channels	Organisational culture
'. . . it stays unclear which factors are the most prominent facilitators or inhibitors of learning and innovation' (Lideway 2004, p. 12)	'Innovation depends on employees who are motivated to contribute to learning and innovative processes in the organization' (Lideway 2004, p. 11)	Climates for initiative and psychological safety are related positively with process innovations and organisational performance (Baer & Frese 2003)	Employees with more supportive managers (Axtell *et al.* 2000)	To encourage collaboration and problem-solving when managing innovation, 'linking mechanisms' can be used, i.e. joint problem-solving teams or matrix organisations; committees and taskforces; project managers and formal meetings (Lideway 2004)	Top management support and involvement; appointment of innovation champion or sponsor; rewards for innovative behaviours and ideas; positive attitude to building on creative ideas, irrespective of their source (Radnor & Robinson 2000)
Most innovations result from a conscious, purposeful search	'Innovation is not the result of an individual and isolated act,	Successful innovation achieved by creating an environment of	Organisational vision and climate for excellence	A culture that fosters and encourages excellent	Organisations need cultures that 'reward and respect the free flow of ideas and

(Continued)

Table 2.1 (Continued)

Innovation attributes	Adopter characteristics	Environmental/context characteristics	Promoter characteristics	Communication channels	Organisational culture
for opportunities (Mohrle & Pannenbacker 1997)	but rather a reality that is constructed socially by different people who make their contributions at different moments in time as the innovation progresses' (Fernández 2001, p. 9)	symbiosis in which leaders help their employees set mutually beneficial ambitions and provide each a forum to achieve them (Amar 2001)	drive 'quality of innovation', whereas participative safety and organisational support drive 'quantity of innovation' (West 1990)	intra-organisational communication to share knowledge is important (Radnor & Robinson 2000)	enquiries' (Amabile 1998, Shalley et al. 2000)
How far it meets customer requirements and targets (Radnor & Robinson 2000)	'...older employees were found to be more innovative. In addition, male employees reported higher	'Organizations with strong egalitarian cultures create a set of norms, symbols and beliefs that encourage learning and	Maintaining an internal awareness of the importance of newness to innovation may end an	Innovation is associated with flows of information across organisational boundaries (Radnor & Robinson 2000)	'...in operational terms, innovation can be translated as an organisation's foresight to "think for the customer" by creating services that

'Encouraging creativity at an individual level will result in improved	'Longer tenure employees showed more positive perceptions of	'Innovation is complex and multi-dimensional in its approach and therefore contextual	Innovation teams comprised of: team leader; innovation
	levels of readiness to innovate – as rated by themselves – than did their female counterparts' (Suliman 2001, p. 49)	innovation in organizations' (Lideway 2004, p. 12)	organisation's innovation efforts. For example, factors such as cultural and structural forces often tend to be impediments to innovation because they lock-in traditional methods and thus shut out new ideas and practices (Miller 1990)

'Building a conducive work climate that facilitates, encourages and supports creativity and

"drive" the market place (offer superior value to the customer)' (Kandampully 2002, p. 19)

Table 2.1 (Continued)

Innovation attributes	Adopter characteristics	Environmental/ context characteristics	Promoter characteristics	Communication channels	Organisational culture
creativity at the level of the group or organisation' (McAdam & McClelland 2002, p. 88)	work climate and higher levels of readiness to innovate' (Suliman 2001, p. 55)	issues will always have to be taken into account for any innovation' (Radnor & Robinson 2000, p. 12)	coach; scouts; innovation strategists; entrepreneur coach and gap managers. (Hellström, et al. 2002)		innovation is critical to the vitality of organisation' (Suliman 2001, p. 50)
Shared vision, participative safety, climate for excellence, practical support (West 1990)		Lack of resource availability is a major block to innovation (Radnor & Robinson 2000)			Successfully innovative organisations develop strategies to cope with the risk of rules preventing the progress of innovative projects (Olin & Wickenberg 2001)

Service innovation described as the 'core competency' of any organisation (Kandampully 2002)

'Organisations should understand that creating a conducive work environment that satisfies the needs of employees is essential for developing their readiness to innovate' (Suliman 2001, p. 57)

The higher the pressure to produce, the lower the readiness to innovate, and vice versa (Benkhoff 1997)

'. . . by emphasising the importance of newness to the process of innovation, managers may identify more targeted interventions that can be used to generate innovativeness more effectively' (Johannessen et al. 2001, p. 28) patient safety. The principal aim is to discover why things go wrong, rectify incorrect actions and make it harder to do the wrong thing again. Couched in this way, action can be perceived as reactive and dialogues as deficit-based. The 'safety solutions' perspective deployed goes through the following stages:

- Understand the patient safety issues.
- Identify areas for solution development.
- Explore possible solutions.
- Test and refine solutions.
- Monitor solutions.

Additionally the NPSA was set up partly in response to the Bristol Royal Infirmary inquiry, which called for a single reporting system for adverse incidents and a culture in which all staff could learn from failures. A major function of the agency has been to collect and analyse information on adverse events from local organisations, NHS staff and patients in order to provide feedback to inform practice. In 2006 the future of the five-year-old NPSA was under review.

What can be learned?

The important reflective question is 'What had it learned?' At a UK conference on patient safety in June 2006, Professor Ian Kennedy said 'wholesale system change' was needed in order to produce recognisable improvements in patient safety. Since then, there has been a flurry of activity. Critical reports have been published from the National Audit Office and the House of Commons Public Accounts Committee. In August 2006, the NPSA's two joint chief executives were sent on 'extended leave'. Articles have been written with evocative titles, such as Lyall's (2006) 'At risk: the safety agency that failed to set the world on fire'. If we view the mission and the subsequent work of the Agency through an r-learning lens, we begin to understand the basis for some of the criticisms cited above and summarised in Table 2.2. In this table, I have juxtaposed the criticisms within the National Audit Office's (2006) publication with the 'change knowledge' derived from the adoption and diffusion of innovation literatures. Table 2.2 shows clearly where more learning was and is necessary.

Learning from change and learning from improvement

Lyall (2006) quotes Professor Kennedy, saying:

> . . . it is hard to escape the conclusion that patchy improvements have been the order of the day. Excellent and important projects have failed to be sustained and incorporated into lasting system improvements.

(Lyall 2006, p. 15)

Table 2.2 Understanding the work of the National Patient Safety Agency through an r-learning lens.

Source of criticism	Nature of criticism	Understanding the criticism through the 'lens of innovation' characteristics
National Audit Office (2006)	Despite improvements in safety culture, many NHS employees still fear blame or unequal treatment if they report incidents, and this remains a major barrier to increasing accurate and honest reporting. There is a need for trusts to re-enforce their commitment to an open and fair reporting culture and to support staffing initiatives to improve. Financial problems and staff shortages can push patient safety down the list of trusts' priorities. Although the potential avoidable costs of patient safety incidents are estimated to be as much as £1 billion, some areas of investment are likely to have a bigger pay back than others	*Relative advantage:* this can be achieved only if an open and fair reporting culture is sustained within organisations. Potential avoidable costs of patient safety incidents need to be effectively communicated. 'The NPSA concentrated on volume data without telling us enough about how we might fix things. I think they could have been more visible in the frontline and given feedback at an earlier stage. The real issue is capturing hearts and minds' (Lyall 2006, p. 15). The report also says that the NPSA is still to demonstrate value for money
	Most trusts analysed incident reports and other information. Indeed, most had been carrying out in-depth investigations of incidents at the local level for a number of years. Seventy-six per cent of trusts told us that they were now encouraging staff to use the NPSA's root cause analysis tool, with many noting that it had helped to improve the quality and consistency of in-depth investigations. A number of trusts remarked that monitoring and investigating incidents created additional	*Compatibility:* there needs to be some constructive alignment between the NPSA's root cause analysis and existing patterns of reporting. High-quality training and support are also required

(Continued)

Table 2.2 (Continued)

Source of criticism	Nature of criticism	Understanding the criticism through the 'lens of innovation' characteristics
	demands on busy senior staff, and consequently they did not always conduct a full root cause analysis of all serious incidents. The quality of reports on investigations was also variable, and recommendations were rarely actioned by organisations outside the trust in which the event had occurred	
	Building a Safer NHS for Patients required the NHS to establish agreed definitions of incidents for the purposes of reporting, gradually moving to an international standardised taxonomy (description and classification of incidents). The NPSA developed its taxonomy in consultation with trusts, but it is unlike many trusts' taxonomies and, in order to link to the national system, trusts had to map it to their own. At the time of our survey, 82 per cent of trusts had had difficulties with the mapping exercise, and 17 per cent of these said that they had experienced major difficulties	*Complexity:* innovations are unlikely to spread and to be sustained if there is confusion with regard to definitions of an incident and the purposes of reporting. 'There was a huge concentration on gathering data, a very complicated collection system, and no quick wins at local level' (Lyall 2006, p. 15)
	To provide evidence that NHS organisations were doing their reasonable best to manage themselves in order to protect patients, staff and the public against risks of all kinds, the Department established the mandatory Controls Assurance Standards in 1999. Trusts had to undertake a self-assessment against defined criteria. For the risk management system	*Trialability:* this is a crucial part of successful uptake and spread, especially where the involvement and participation of patients is concerned

standard, these criteria included board accountability, adverse incident reporting and complaints and claims handling. Over the five years of its operation, average compliance increased from 52 per cent to 87 per cent

Patients have little involvement in the identification of patient safety priorities and in the design of solutions in most trusts

Under-reporting is a problem in some staff groups more than others, and there is a perception among staff that not all employees take responsibility for patient safety reporting

As nine out of ten NHS employees work in teams, effective communication between staff is important to reduce the risk of unintended harm to patients, and yet trusts often cite failure in communication as a reason for an incident. Communicating openly with patients and carers is also essential, but only 24 per cent of trusts were routinely informing patients when an incident that they had been involved in was reported to the trust

Dissemination of learning and the development of solutions were patchy, and there was also no systematic monitoring to ensure implementation within the trust

Observability: we know that an important component of successful diffusions of innovations is to keep the process and the learning visible. Difficulties will always occur in uptake and spread when this ceases to happen. For example, Lyall (2006, p. 14) writes: 'Doctors were less likely than other groups of staff to report incidents and doubts remain among healthcare workers as to whether the agency can really make a difference. Some believe that lack of visibility and demonstrable effectiveness at local level mean the agency has essentially failed'

Professor Kennedy also said that sustainable improvements at the frontline were not yet embedded. We need to engage in some serious reflection on the NPSA's view of how we might best learn from adverse incidents. Additionally, we might think again about the title of the National Audit Office's report (2006), which contains the word 'learning'. But what conception(s) of learning are being used here? I suggest that two fundamental issues emerge from the NPSA case. First, we need to learn and appropriately apply knowledge from the diffusion of innovation literatures. This is necessary if we are to achieve a goal of 'wholesale system change'. Second, we need a deep appreciation of how we can best learn from established and emerging 'change knowledge'. This is necessary if we are to make wise and ethical decisions concerning patient safety. The characteristics of r-learning suggested in this book may play a part in understanding the issues that have confronted the NPSA (see Fig. 0.2). For example, r-learning (reflective learning) enables us to:

Develop appreciations

I suggest that we should not always ask 'What are the barriers to reducing patient safety incidents?' but 'What are successful (gateway) systems for patient safety?', 'What are the root causes of these successes?' and 'How can we grow in the direction of success?' Here I am emphasising the power of the positive question. These generate strength-based, not deficit-based, conversations – conversations that have the potential to be more uplifting, energising and hopeful. I am not saying that adverse incidents and 'problems' should not be reflected upon and action taken. What I am proposing is that if we concentrate on our successes, then we naturally grow in that direction. In doing so, the problems tend to get squeezed out over time. The goal is the same, namely to build a safe healthcare system. It is the process that is different, perhaps a more successful and lasting one. There is a strong suggestion in the case of the NPSA, as described above, that one process (the NPSA's safety solutions perspective) has not achieved sustainable improvements. Maybe another process might be tried. The Institute of Medicine (1999, p. 2) puts it this way:

> Mistakes can best be prevented by designing the health system at all levels to make it safer, to make it harder for people to do something wrong and easier for them to do it right. Of course, this does not mean that individuals can be careless. People must be vigilant and held responsible for their actions. But when an error occurs, blaming an individual does little to make the system safer and prevent someone else from committing the same error.

Later we read:

> It may be part of human nature to err; but it is also part of human nature to create solutions, find better alternatives and meet the challenges ahead.

(Institute of Medicine 1999, p. 6)

A key phrase is designing a system where it is easier to do things right than wrong. Focusing on what's right, what's going well and the root causes of 'rightness' and 'wellness' is a positive start.

Re-frame experience

In general I suggest the NPSA case reminds us that we must pay even closer attention to our own and others' powerful inclinations to prioritise working with and from problems. The criticism of NPSA regarding 'no quick wins at local level' (Lyall 2006, p. 15) confronts us with a challenge: that it is often unwise to simply be preoccupied with the immediate relief of today's problems and to pursue only behavioural strategies that bring about short-term solutions. If we do, we are in danger of taking our eye off the deeper, underlying changes that need to be made in achieving better patient safety. In a strange way, short-termism has the effect of doing exactly what we need to avoid: it actually works to prevent, not support, sustainable improvement. Kegan & Lahey (2001, p. 43) put it this way:

> . . . strange as it may sound, even though something is surely gained when a problem is solved, something is also lost. For one thing, we lose a problem. 'But that's the point!' the conscientious professional responds. 'What could be wrong with having one less problem?' Our reply is that, without doubt, many problems may need only to be solved, but if we regard all our problems as bugs in the system, the best we will ever do in removing them is preserve the system – and it [the system] may be responsible for producing the bugs in the first place! When we solve a problem quickly, the one thing we can usually be certain of is that we ourselves are the same people coming out of the problem as we are going into it.

Focus upon success

So what can we do? One practical thing is to re-frame the problems of practice and instead look at successes, focus on them and learn more about sustaining them. By doing this, we may be sustaining a system that produces what we want rather than what we don't want. If this sounds too idealistic, then at least we could try to look at 'promising practices' – those that give us a sense of optimism that, if enacted, give ourselves a chance of improving what we do. To re-frame around success requires a change in the language(s) we use to describe our work. So it follows that we need to know who the language and discourse-shaping leaders are in our healthcare organisation, those who have the opportunity and influence to alter (negatively) habitual and often favoured ways of talking about practice. Instead of talking about what we want less of (problems), we might talk about what we want more of (successes). Instead of using the languages of complaint, disappointment and resignation ('things will never change around here'), we try to use the languages of hope, optimism and commitment more often.

Build individual and collective wisdom

At an international Royal College of Nursing Practice development conference (Practice Development, Action Research and Reflective Practice:
6th International Conference – Enhancing Practice 6: Innovation, Creativity,
Patient Care and Professionalism, 18–20 October 2006, Heriot-Watt
University, Edinburgh, UK), I presented a 90-minute workshop on reflective learning. During this workshop I asked the 30 participants to think
about their answer to the question 'What sorts of things, if they were to
happen more frequently in your clinical area, would you experience as
being more supportive and appreciative of you and your work?' I asked
the participants to try not to edit their responses through the usual filters
of possibility or likelihood. After some minutes of thought, the general
themes to emerge were about people and behaviours – people speaking
to each other differently, and overt and noticeable behaviours that demonstrated support and appreciation. These themes were inferred through
phrases such as 'We don't really talk to each other – more about each
other' and 'Nothing really changes. We talk about what we want and
need, to do a good job, but we usually end up going round and round
talking about the same old problems. Nothing ever seems to change.' In
general, participants reported that it was harder to think about this question than one I offered later, namely, 'What sorts of things, if they were to
happen less frequently in your clinical area, would you experience as
being more supportive and appreciative of you and your work?' Here,
there were a flood of responses around, for example, a reduction in
excessive workloads, less paperwork, less bitching and running each
other down, less staff turnover, less duplication, less resentment, less
weariness, and so on.

What were we learning?

First, we learned that these comments were being articulated by people
who had a good memory of the different ways they experienced their
nursing work. Second, we were all well-practised in using languages that
focused on what we want less of (problems), rather than what we want
more of (success and satisfaction). For some, a discourse about problems
was regarded as almost second nature. Third, in many healthcare organisations, the language of problems (and its associated languages of risk
management, root cause analysis, and so on) was felt to be more noticeable and audible than the language of success. Finally, we learned that getting trapped in deficit-based conversations (addressing what we do not
have, rather than focusing on what we have) does not really transform and
improve anything. Usually these conversations never go anywhere, like
the quote above from a workshop participant suggests: just 'round and
round'. They become an end in themselves. Such conversations may allow
staff to let off steam, which may be important. Additionally, providing a
space for staff to feel less alone in their unhappiness or disappointment

may also be helpful, especially if allies who share such concerns and experiences are found. In the end, it might boil down to this. How far should we try to build collective practice wisdom from a shared and deep understanding of the root causes of our success or of our failings and failures?

Demonstrate achievement

Issues around patient safety, near-misses, safety incidents and risk management, among others, can be linked closely with the languages of blame and responsibility. What went wrong and who is responsible? Whose fault is it? Patient safety is a complex world. There are many people and interactions that contribute to the way things are. Therefore, it is important to develop positive workplace habits that support staff to collectively reflect upon the question 'What are we doing that enables us to achieve the best we can?' This is a very different question from the more commonly asked (or felt) question 'What is happening that is inhibiting us from being the best we can?' Busyness and taking on too many commitments are common inhibiting influences. Being unable to say 'no' and an inability to delegate, when appropriate, are two further inhibiters. Responding to the latter question is not about humiliating or diminishing ourselves. It is not about our shortcomings or limitations. It has more to do with trying to articulate some kind of positive response to it and trying to learn from this. Responding positively is a form of responsibility. In a reflective organisation, there are opportunities for asking and responding to such questions. Learning from the enabling or inhibiting behaviours we identify is an example of responsible action.

The risk of quick wins

Demonstrable achievement couched in terms of quick wins may be clinically significant, but pressures like this do involve risk: the risk of not learning the lesson. Removing the problem is one kind of achievement; another is sticking with some problems. This is not as crazy as it may sound. Solving and removing the problem from the system may be a desirable outcome. But the real lesson to be learned may be from the system itself. It is a matter of careful judgement as to which problems may be worth sticking with. The point I am making is that a mindset of simply removing problems from the healthcare system, as fast as possible, may be a short-lived gain. For example, a senior healthcare manager told me that she had rushed (for a number of reasons) into undertaking some work to try to improve her hospital's outpatient department, which was receiving an increasing number of patient complaints and suffering from increasing staff sickness rates. Her hastiness was fuelled by her genuine belief that it was important and necessary to pay attention and respond to patient complaints. Her passion for service improvement came across to others. Always, where there is such passion, there are possibilities for service improvement. In her mind, quick wins became equated with responding to the complaints she was receiving. Her answer was to make a plan to restructure the department. In her rush, she kept to a minimum the number of occasions for consultation with all stakeholders and paid a considerable amount of money, to an external agency, to help her implement her plan, fast. Initially, things seemed to be better. The restructuring of the department meant that she heard fewer complaints. But then something worrying began to happen. After six months, she began to receive more complaints – more complaints than before. The problem had not gone away.

In discussion with her, we began to re-frame what evidence of 'demonstrating achievement' might look like. In her rush for quick wins, she forgot to reflect upon other people's experience of a similar improvement process and even lessons learned from within her own hospital. By concentrating on reducing complaints as fast as possible, she lost the chance to bring a revitalising energy into the outpatient department. Admittedly this would have taken more time, but it might have been time well spent. Re-structuring and re-positioning staff into new teams was not the solution to her problem. She forgot the lesson that sustainable service improvement, in this case, would stand a better chance of success if she had managed to re-frame tackling patient complaints, by transforming this into a deeper appreciation of staff commitments. Stemming the tide of complaints was not the root cause of a successful department; understanding staff commitments, hopes and concerns first and then acting appropriately was. Engaging in conversations with all staff about what they wanted their outpatient department to stand for was the root of success. Understanding their convictions was. Regarding a complaint not as a signal of what was wrong but as a signal of what a patient really cared about was. Instead of trying to engage in fewer conversations of complaint, on reflection she began to feel that she may have done better if she had focused on engaging in more conversations about commitment. In a lengthy reflective conversation, she developed her appreciation that she could have powerfully demonstrated achievement had she been able to facilitate an observable shift in the mindset of staff, and one away from the dominant language of complaint within the department. A new structure did not do the trick, as habitual patterns of behaviour and the ways staff conversed with each other did not change. A new structure masked underlying patterns of interaction that were still fuelled by disappointment, cynicism, wishing and complaint. An opportunity missed was in not seeing and believing that the root cause of service success was in staff experiencing themselves as committed people holding particular convictions that needed to be better understood. Additionally, there were missed opportunities for staff to air their convictions – those that they felt were personally significant and patient sensitive and, in doing so, that were most deserving of being promoted and defended. The healthcare manager is now re-framing this initiative and planning ways to engage in a different kind of conversation with stakeholders involved in the outpatient department.

How do we change the way we talk to each other?

Kegan & Lahey (2001) explore this idea of how we might change the way we talk to each other in their book that sets out different languages for workplace transformation. Two of their languages relevant to the example above and to healthcare service development in general are the characteristics of a language of blame and of a language of personal responsibility.

Kegan & Lahey juxtapose the characteristics to enable comparisons to be made. For example, holding others responsible for gaps between intentions and reality (blaming) is set alongside expressing personal responsibility for behaviours that may contribute to such gaps. Another example is the way a characteristic of a language of blame is associated with questions for others to answer. A characteristic of a language of personal responsibility is associated with raising questions for oneself to answer.

Root cause analysis

In the case of the NPSA, many trusts were using their root cause analysis tool, and yet many NHS employees still feared blame and unequal treatment if they reported incidents. The best incident report forms count for nothing if 'only 24% of trusts were routinely informing patients when an incident, that they had been involved in, was reported to the trust' (National Audit Office 2006, p. 4). Agreeing the definitions of incidents for the purpose of reporting is pointless if the dissemination of learning and the development of solutions is patchy (see Table 2.2). The sobering lesson from this is that creating more knowledge, and seeing this as an achievement, is no guarantee of bringing us closer to solutions. It carries with it no guarantee that we can get to the root causes of success. We need to break out of the vicious cycle of doing more of the same, only harder. What happens if more of the same ways of working, but harder, yields only more of the same? Sometimes the questions we ask and the ways we pursue them actually prevent the very thing we strive for. They prevent learning and improvement. Maybe how we talk to each other and formulate frame-shifting questions are good places to begin our search for success. Maybe changing the way we talk can change the way we work?

West (1990, p. 90) lists the following characteristics of workgroups when they are striving to create something new and innovative:

- *Vision:* The group needs to have a clear focus or goal negotiated and shared by the group, valued within the group and regarded as attainable (see also Peters and Waterman 1982).
- *Participative safety:* The group needs to work in a non-threatening context that provides sufficient 'space' (emotional, mental, physical) to allow members to participate fully in decision-making.
- *Climate of excellence in task performance:* Here, 'climate' means a working context that expects and welcomes feedback and evaluation around issues of quality.

- *Practical support:* The organisation provides real and tangible support to the work group.

In this book, we are thinking about what makes an innovation, such as r-learning, successful system-wide. King & Anderson (1995) identified the following factors that address this:

- A democratic, collaborative leadership style that encourages and motivates team members. I take up this notion of leadership qualities later (see p. 190).
- Cohesiveness between team members. A heterogeneous team is an advantage for idea generation in order to avoid 'groupthink', but King & Anderson suggest that a homogeneous team is desirable for smooth implementation.

These are complicated ideas to work with. What is a homogeneous or heterogeneous team? Are we talking about what staff know and can do? Is it about difference and diversity with regard to values, experience or discipline? Is it about roles, responsibilities, flexibility or adaptiveness? Is it cohesiveness as perceived by those within the team (or workgroup, network, etc.), or by those outside of the team? These perceptions could be very different. Let me offer you an illustration of this.

Facilitating r-learning at the centre of a cancer care network

A strategic framework for improving cancer services was being developed for a large urban area in the UK. It was being jointly led by the Strategic Health Authority and the cancer network for that area. The aim of the framework was to bring together, into a cohesive whole, service development plans that, until recently, had evolved in relative isolation. More specifically and urgently a need was felt to develop plans for supportive and palliative care (SPC), which responded positively to the National Institute of Clinical Excellence (NICE) national standards for improving clinical outcomes. The intention was to make the SPC plan an integral part of the strategic framework. A baseline assessment of current provision was undertaken, which provided useful data in order to map out services, activities and resources currently provided across the network. The cancer network team met with NHS trust managers, lead clinicians and user representatives. Data around capacity planning, workforce (recruitment and retention of staff), multidisciplinary teamworking, new information and communication technology (ICT) requirements, managing risks, and so on, was gathered. This work took up the best part of two years.

At the point where the SPC data were being integrated with other cancer services data to form a coherent, cost-effective and NICE-responsive plan, the cancer network team of 15 people thought it prudent to begin a process of systematic, evidence-based r-learning. At the heart of this commitment was a need to better understand two questions:

- How well do *we* see ourselves working as a cancer network team?
- How do *others* regard us as a cancer network team?

A reflective conversation

As a catalyst for a reflective conversation about the first question, all team members were invited to complete an online version of a team culture questionnaire called STEPs (Institute of Reflective Practice UK 2007). This asks individuals within a group or team to respond to 50 statements concerned with their perceptions of working with each other. The results are shown in Fig. 2.3. This conversation was further enriched by data

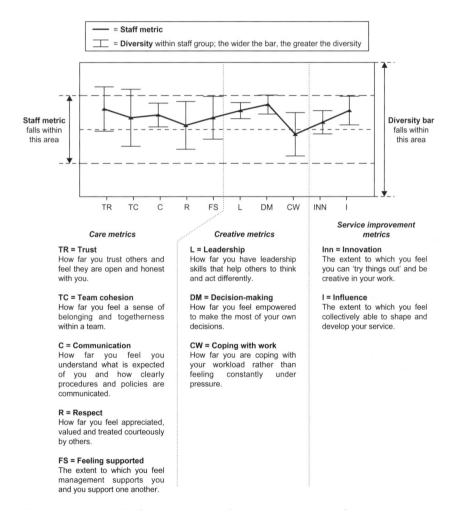

Figure 2.3 Results from a team culture questionnaire for a cancer network team.

from a second questionnaire made up of statements on which the cancer team members wished to receive feedback. They were sent out to 15 key players in cancer care in acute primary care trusts and hospices within the reach of the network. All 15 key players completed and returned the questionnaire online.

The development and implementation of a strategic framework for improving cancer services had at its core a team of highly motivated and skilful practitioners who were committed to r-learning. They were developing an innovative plan that Halladay & Bero (2000) would regard as a 'systemic re-orientation'. In their terms, this is an:

> . . . attempt to alter the fabric and structure of the system in which health care is provided. It involves the re-conception of the task as one taking place within a holistic system of care, inclusive of health care organisations, universities, professional bodies, patient groups, payers and regulators.

(Halladay & Bero 2000, p. 44)

Figure 2.3 shows the results of the cancer network team's STEPs questionnaire. There are two 'stories' within the box. The first story relates to the uneven line. This represents the whole team's (consensual) view around each of the ten metrics (measures) associated with care, creativity and service improvement. The other story is illustrated by the series of bars associated with each of the metrics. The greater the width of the bar, the greater the diversity of view, within the team, associated with that particular metric.

The STEPs results and the graph of external perceptions were presented to the team, with some explanation of their visual portrayal by IRP-UK staff. Below is how the conversation unfurled. See if you can hear the way the conversation begins in deficit-based mode, develops into a much more strength-based and optimistic conversation, and concludes by sliding back a little into 'fixing' deficits. The conversation also makes the point that the cancer team thought they were all very much 'on the same page' and homogeneous with regard to service development, in King & Anderson's (1995) terms. There is evidence in Figs 2.3 and 2.4 that leads us to question this. One clue to understanding this is the substantial degree of diversity (width of the bars) shown in Fig. 2.3.

Laura: Oh dear! We're obviously not coping very well with our workloads are we?
Sue: Now there's a surprise! We didn't need a graph to tell us that did we?
Paul: And not only are we struggling with work, but we don't have time to reflect on it and make any changes.

Laura: And because of too much work and no time to reflect, there's no way we can try different ways of working or 'be creative', as it says here.
Sue: I wish!
James: So, overall, not a pretty picture, if you excuse the pun.
Sue: That's why I don't see the point of sessions like this. We just get told what we already know, and I get even more depressed than I already am.

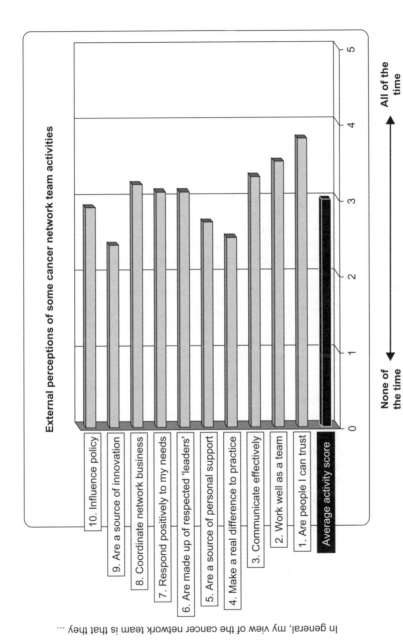

Figure 2.4 Some external perceptions of the cancer network team.

Laura: At least we only fall below the middle line in one category – the coping with work one.

Mary: Yes, but isn't that the most important one? If we're not managing our workloads, then it impacts on everything else.

Jacqui: But does it? Why aren't all the scores below the middle line then?

Sue: Well, they nearly all are.

Jacqui: That's a bit judgemental, Sue. No, they're not. To be fair, we have got some scores nearer the top line – like trust and decision-making. That must be good news?

Paul: But not really surprising – the decision-making point, that is. We have to make our own decisions because of the type of team that we are. Basically we're autonomous, aren't we?

Laura: And I would expect us to trust each other, or our network would fall apart.

Mary: Seems strange, then, that our team cohesion and communication aren't much higher.

Laura: Not only that: look at the difference we have in opinion! Some of us think team cohesion is well high and some think it's way down.

Sue: I know where my point would be.

Jacqui: Maybe that's the problem, Sue? We don't communicate with each other as much as we should, so we don't get a feeling of being part of a team as much as we could.

Paul: But you can't communicate more when you're struggling to cope with the work, so it's a catch-22 – again.

Laura: But some of us think we're coping with work a lot better than others.

Mary: So, what's the secret, please?

Sue: Yes, own up! Who's letting the team down and actually thinks we haven't got enough work to do?

James: Maybe if our 'feeling supported' point was higher, we'd have a higher score for coping with work too?

Paul: Well, that's a resource issue isn't it?

Laura: No, I don't think it's as complicated as that. Someone just saying 'thank you' or 'I really appreciated what you did for that person' would be enough for me. I don't need an hour every week having therapy.

Paul: I didn't mean that, Laura. It's just that lack of time and people feeling under pressure makes it difficult to even notice what anyone else is doing.

Mary: Back to my team cohesion and communication point. The question is: how do we make time?

Sue: We can't.

Jacqui: Hang on! We're just going round in circles and the conversation's going a bit negative, which is a shame because I do actually like my work and I like this team.

[general agreement]

Facilitator: Perhaps it might be timely to look at what the 'External perceptions' graph tells you? It might help you to look at your own portrait a bit differently?

Sue: Or get more depressed.

Paul: I think Sue's going to take some convincing.

[team looks at External perceptions graph]

Mary: OK, as I seem to have got hung up on team cohesion and communication, I think we should pat ourselves on the back because the majority of people in our wider network say we work well as a team and we communicate effectively.

Paul: So we must be making a pretty good impression, even if we don't feel it ourselves. We do it for them, but are we doing it enough within our team?

Jacqui: But that's exactly where I think we've been too hard on ourselves. We could read our own portrait in a much more positive way than we have done. I think we should be really pleased with the level of trust that we have in this team, and I'm even happier that the wider network think we're a team who they can really trust.

James: And it's making me wonder whether it's not such a bad thing to have the diversity in the team in some areas. We'd be a pretty boring bunch if the blue line was dead flat across the top and the pink bars were on top of each other.

Mary: *Boring, but brilliant!*

[laughter]

Laura: That would make a nice change.

Jacqui: I actually like the way the portrait gives highs and lows. I can see myself trying to change one of the points and seeing if it affects another. Like Mary's 'communication' point. If I make more effort in communicating with just one other person in the team, I think the 'feeling supported' would rise too.

Mary: And that has to affect team cohesion.

Paul: So we've shifted three of the care metrics up in one go.

Laura: And maybe that would influence the 'coping with work' bit?

Mary: Which gives us more time to try new things.

Sue: God, now you are getting carried away. It's never going to work like that, or we would all have done it ages ago.

Jacqui: But would we? This is the first time I've ever talked about some of these issues, and it's made me realise how much I don't know about some people in this team. I'd love to change that.

[general agreement]

Facilitator: It might be an appropriate time, then, to ask a question about what you're really proud of, a success, something you want to do more of in order to move the team even further forward.

Paul: Couldn't we all put that question on the table?

Facilitator: Absolutely. Why not?

Jacqui: Maybe take it in turns, then, and briefly give our thoughts on where the team is now and where we'd like it to be this time next year?

Paul: Or sooner!

Jacqui: So can I start with what I think we are doing well, despite the constraints? Because I think that every member of this team puts others first and tries to give them the best service they possibly can. That's something we should be proud of and celebrate. And how do I see the team moving forward? Well, we know there are aspects of the service that we can still improve, so I suggest we identify one thing as a team which we can jointly agree on and then find ways to make it happen.

Laura: I think we need more opportunities like this to keep in touch with each other. I hardly ever meet up with some people in this team, which seems crazy because we all need each other to make the service work.

Mary: We've probably talked more, and listened to each other more, during this session than over the last month.

Paul: Now, that is a resource issue. What's it cost the service to give us a day's training like this one?

Laura: But isn't it worth it? I'd rather spend some quality time with everyone in one place, now and again, than get piles of emails or grab snippets of information from telephone calls and Post-Its.

Jacqui: So build in more time to work together as a team?

Laura: Yes, please.

Mary: But, keep the day focused like this one, have a realistic agenda – and lunch, please!

James: I liked Jacqui's earlier suggestion: find a way to communicate better with just one other person in this team and see the knock-on effects.

Paul: And how do you define 'communication'?

Jacqui: Understanding each other's needs and expectations. Listening to each other and appreciating what we want from one another.

Sue: Say we can't give what the other one wants?

Jacqui: It may be enough that you've listened. You may be surprised at what others' expectations are.

Facilitator: So, some protected time to meet and reflect? And better communication with at least one other person within the team? What other suggestions would you like to add?

Paul: To be honest, I'd rather stick to those two. If the list gets too long, it will defeat the object. It will all get a bit messy.

[general agreement]

Facilitator: OK. So, let's sum up this conversation on that positive note and, hopefully, Jacqui will be able to sort out a date in the diary for a follow-up session in the not too distant future?

Jacqui: No problem. Will do!

What can we learn from this?

What are some of the important things we can learn from this conversation?

- Some members of the team seem, on this occasion, to have a predilection for more deficit-based, problem-oriented contributions. These can sound negative to colleagues. They are contributions more about 'can't do' rather than 'can do'. Sue's words are an example of this:
  + 'Now there's a surprise! We didn't need a graph to tell us that did we?'
  + 'Yes, own up! Who's letting the team down and actually thinks we haven't got enough work to do?'
  + 'We can't.'
  + 'Or get more depressed.'
  + 'God, now you are getting carried away. It's never going to work like that, or we would all have done it ages ago.'
  + 'Say we can't give what the other one wants?'

- On the other hand, we can find more positive, optimistic, strength-based and uplifting comments. Jacqui's contributions are an example of this. She is also the team leader. For example:
  + 'Hang on! We're just going round in circles and the conversation's going a bit negative, which is a shame because I do actually like my work and I like this team.'
  + 'But that's exactly where I think we've been too hard on ourselves. We could read our own portrait in a much more positive way than we have done. I think we should be really pleased with the level of trust that we have in this team, and I'm even happier that the wider network think we're a team who *they* can really trust.'
- Through this r-learning conversation, team members came to appreciate that there was a far greater degree of diversity within the team (heterogeneity) than they had thought. Importantly, the conversation begins to suggest that it was not the differences between them that were problematic, but the judgements they made about each other.
- In order to build more success, they had to become even better listeners to each other, to how others felt, to what others were thinking.
- They needed more time to think and reflect.
- There was an acknowledgement that moving forward, as a team, to develop the strategic framework for improving cancer services was likely to be a bit messy at times. But 'reality doesn't change itself. We need to act' (Wheatley 2002, p. 51).
- R-learning conversations like the one above really need to be evidence-enriched. Kitson *et al.* (1998) developed an equation that helps us see some of the connections between evidence and the successful implementation, or use of it. I have taken the liberty of changing the F in their equation $SI = f(E, C, F)$ to T – that is, from $F =$ facilitation to $T =$ team. Their equation makes us think about the coverage of an uptake of an innovation in this way: $SI = f(E, C, T)$ where, SI (successful implementation of an idea/innovation) is a function (f) of the relationship between E (evidence):
  + the research (questionnaire) findings;
  + clinical experience (of the cancer network team);
  + patient (user) preferences;

C *(context)*:
- an understanding of the prevailing cultures within the acute primary care trusts and hospices;
  + the nature of human relationships within the cancer network;
  + the cancer network team's approach to supporting and developing services;

T *(team)*:
  + the gifts, talents and aspirations of individual network team members;
  + the characteristics of the SPC steering group;

♦ the knowledge, skills and sensitivities of the SPC steering group and working group chairs (leaders).

• In more general terms, the coverage and uptake of an innovation such as r-learning are intimately tied up with the kinds of language we use. When working in cultures of disappointment, cynicism and blame, a comment such as 'I wish!' takes on a very different meaning than when used in a team, and within a healthcare organisation, where there is a more appreciative and optimistic mindscape. In Table 2.3, I use some of the statements from the cancer network team conversation, and add other comments. I try to show how the pervasive culture(s) within our work teams and organisations affect how we 'hear' each statement. Organisational cultures wash over us and cause us to filter information in and out of our sensory receptors in particular ways.

R-learning in a paediatric intensive care unit

Most of the content of Table 2.3 was developed during an appreciative r-learning day with a group of staff from a paediatric intensive care unit. On a flipchart, I wrote with a large marker pen 'blame culture'. This caused some spontaneous 'I know what you mean'-type comments. Next to this I wrote, 'appreciative culture'. This generated a few nervous laughs and some not-so-quiet 'um's. The staff had not come across workplace cultures described in this way before. On the line below, I wrote the statement 'You will do better next time'. Underneath 'blame culture' I wrote 'threat' and under 'appreciative culture' I wrote 'encouragement'. On the next line, I wrote 'I didn't expect you to do it that way'. This time under blame, I wrote 'reprimand' and under appreciation 'opinion'. This generated much discussion. I then progressively added to the list of

Table 2.3 From blame to appreciation.

Statement	Blame culture	Appreciative culture
'You will do better next time'	Threat	Encouragement
'I didn't expect you to do it that way'	Reprimand	Opinion
'You need to take a break'	Order	Concern
'I haven't seen it done like that before'	Contempt	Interest
'Well that's certainly a different approach to tackling the problem'	Sarcasm	Observation
'Let's wait and see, shall we?'	Dismissive	Curiosity
'Why have you done it like that?'	Accusation	Enquiry
'I know what to do'	Control	Reassurance
'It would certainly help if you read up on that'	Frustration	Invitation
'Just watch me, I'll show you how to do it'	Annoyance	Demonstration

statements. In pairs, staff discussed the different ways the statement might be 'heard' in these two contrasting cultures.

What can we learn from this?

There are a number of lessons to be drawn from this example. First, the dominant workplace culture or organisational mindscape has a major impact on our perception. If we feel that we are working in a blame culture, we will hear the words from that frame. The two statements might have been meant as words of encouragement or opinion, but this is probably not the way they will be heard. Second, the prevailing organisational mindscape encourages and even approves of certain kinds of behaviour. If everyone feels they are working in a blame culture, it is much more likely that staff will behave in blaming ways. We often find ourselves growing in the direction that is taking most of our energy and attention. Similarly, if we believe we work in an appreciative culture, staff are more likely to behave in supportive and forgiving ways. Third, organisational cultures can be hard to shift and change. They can be self-sustaining. For example, because I hear the words 'You will do better next time' as a threat, I have a tendency to accept them as proof that I do indeed work in a blame culture. And then what might follow? 'Did you hear that? She just threatened me. She's bullying me. That's so typical of the way things are around here!' We get caught up in a vicious spiral of blaming language and blaming behaviours.

What do we know about scaling up?

The World Health Organization (2004) explores the idea of *rapid scale-up* and draws upon the Institute for Healthcare Improvement's (2003) Breakthrough Series Collaborative Model to illustrate how this might work. Many of the lessons learned, if taken on face value, appear to be applicable to the process of scaling up r-learning. For example, rapid scale-up might occur if:

- adoption takes place in multiple sites, simultaneously. So we don't have one group of 'early adopters' but a number of groups, not one 'champion' but a number of 'champions';
- we think about it as a simultaneous rather than a sequential process;
- there is a culture of knowledge-sharing among peers, with the various factors influencing success being documented;
- we understand the notion of 'tipping point' (see p. 163). All diffusions of innovation have a tipping point. Beyond this point, diffusion becomes increasingly difficult to stop. The skill is knowing how to reach the innovation's tipping point and what behaviours lead to this;
- it is seen as an iterative process of trying to repeat the processes leading to local success, with more and more staff groups. However, this requires an appreciation of the influence of local, contextual factors.

In this book I define the scaling up of r-learning as an activity of increasing the access to, uptake of and impact on more and more people, over time, across a healthcare organisation, and thereby transforming reflection from an individualistic practice into a self-sustaining, collective learning process.

What are some of the challenges to scaling up?

Let's begin with the phrase 'rate of adoption', which is clearly linked with the speed with which r-learning is scaled up. Individual healthcare staff and teams adopt different innovations (of which r-learning may be perceived as one example) and spread them at different rates to other individuals and teams. Some new, 'good' or fashionable ideas are never adopted. Rogers (1983, 1995) and Rogers & Scott (1997) suggest that there are a number of important elements in what they call the *innovation-decision process* that we should bear in mind. First, there is the time it takes from staff becoming aware of the nature and benefits of r-learning, to forming an opinion about it. This opinion-forming element is a critical phase in the whole process. In my experience, this can take anything from minutes to months. Second, there is the time involved in deciding to scale it up, delay it or prioritise something else. This may involve the time it takes to think about how to marshal your argument, lobby for support or present at committees or the trust board, preparing a business case, linking the outcomes of r-learning to trust targets, dovetailing it into ongoing work for the Healthcare Commission's annual health check, organising presentations from those early adopters in the organisation who have some positive experiences to share, and so on. Third, there is the time involved in implementing r-learning once the decision has been made to scale it up. This has a great deal to do with the 'culture of innovation' within the organisation, which I will come back to later. A fourth element is the existing patterns of behaviours among staff and how far engaging fully in r-learning entails these patterns changing in some way. Finally there is the role played by the *critical mass*. In scaling up r-learning so that it becomes an organisation-wide collective work process, the goal is to try to create a critical mass of adopters so that further spread becomes a self-sustaining process. When this critical mass is reached, it might be regarded as the 'tipping point' (Gladwell 2005). Additionally, in Fig. 2.2 I use the notion of 'readiness' for scaling up when an organisation's espoused values (in relation to r-learning) seem to fit well with existing patterns of behaviour.

Readiness for innovation

Greenhalgh *et al.* (2004) place this in the broad context of a 'system's readiness for innovation' and ask 'What steps must be taken by service organisations when moving towards a state of readiness (i.e. with all players on board and with protected time and funding), and how can this overall process be supported and enhanced?' Additionally they ask:

- How can innovation fit best be assessed?
- How can the implications of the innovation be assessed and fed into the decision-making process?
- What measures enhance the success of efforts to secure funding from the innovation in the resource-allocation cycle?
- How can the organisation's capacity to evaluate the impact of the innovation be enhanced?
- What are the characteristics of organisations that successfully avoid taking up 'bad ideas'? Are they just lucky, or do they have better mechanisms for evaluating the ideas and anticipating the subsequent effects? (Greenhalgh *et al.* 2004)

Getting things right

The World Bank (2004) offers us an interesting and compelling summary of the lessons it has learned about scaling up. Their 'four messages' are extremely relevant to making a good response to this book's central question (see p. 5). I have summarised and applied the messages thus:

Message 1 **Get the politics right**
In other words, spend time fostering commitment, a culture of learning and an attitude that turns adversity into a window of opportunity. Those responsible for scaling up need to have good micro-political skills.

Message 2 **Keep the focus on staff**
The scaling up of r-learning will work only if staff want it to succeed. Staff participation and feelings of ownership are crucial here.

Message 3 **Get the implementation right**
We don't have to think everything through in detail. But successful scaling up does depend upon a mindset of continuous learning from what's working well.

Message 4 **Get the support for innovation right**
It is worth spending time building up a significant 'interest group' who not only start the process but also have the power and influence to embed and sustain the process, over time, within the organisation.

Adoption as a staged process: the work of Rogers (1983, 1995)

Just as we found stage thinking in action step 1 when discussing 'models of reflection', we find it again in innovation-adoption thinking. Wolfe (1994) identified as many as ten stages. Rogers' work has been influential in describing the way innovations tend to be adopted in organisations.

He proposed a five-stage model of the process of adoption. These stages are:

Stage 1   Knowledge
This is where the individual, team or other decision-making unit is exposed to and begins to understand the nature and purpose of the innovation. Johannessen *et al.* (2001) suggest that 'newness' is the essence of an innovation. This confirms Slappendel's (1996) view that innovation is something more than simply change. After a while, an innovation may become firmly embedded within the organisation, may lose its perceived 'newness' and be seen much more as a routine (Cooper & Zmud 1990).

Stage 2   Persuasion
This is an opinion-forming stage where the decision-makers develop a favourable or unfavourable view of the innovation. Some criteria used for this are specified on p. 129. It is not the innovation per se that's important. What matters is the value of the innovation (e.g. of r-learning) as perceived by staff (Kandampully 2002).

Stage 3   Decision
This is the point, after due process, when the decision-makers decide whether or not to adopt the innovation.

Stage 4   Implementation
Here, the innovation is put into practice.

Stage 5   Confirmation
After implementation, the decision-makers seek some positive signs and reinforcement that their decision to adopt (or not) was a prudent one.

Rogers' S-curve

In much of the literature on the adoption of innovations we find reference to Rogers' S-curve (Rogers 1995). This describes the adoption of innovations through a particular population (e.g. a workforce). Rogers' S-curve was developed from studying the uptake of a hybrid corn variety among farmers in an Iowan county. This initial study has been replicated for many other innovations. The study found that the adoption process had an S-shape. More generally, Rogers found this to be true when numbers of adopters were plotted against time. In essence, the S-curve model shows that any innovation is first adopted by a few people within the organisation. As more people use it and others see it being used, it is adopted more widely – but this happens only if the innovation is perceived as being 'better' than what went before. Once the adoption of the innovation reaches the level of a critical mass of adopters, it proceeds rapidly. At some point, the innovation reaches those parts of the workforce that are less likely, for whatever reason, to adopt it. Rogers labels the characteristics of these different kinds of adopter thus: 'Innovators', 'Early adopters', 'Early majority', 'Late majority' and 'Laggards'.

There are many contextual factors that serve to modify, distort or even refute the tidy impression that the S-curve gives. We must not forget that a healthcare organisation is a social system, and so there are many things that help and hinder the process of adoption. Much of this is concerned with the cultures within the organisation, for example the extent to which there is a culture of innovation already in existence, a culture of support where staff are helped to try out new things and not blamed if the innovation does not seem to be fulfilling its promise, a culture of learning where staff groups meet to share their thoughts and feelings about an innovation, and so on. Other reasons affecting the rate of adoption may be associated with the appointment of those chosen to lead the innovation, such as project managers, the availability of any funds necessary to put the innovation into practice, the way any resistance is managed constructively, and the way space is created so that staff have the time, among everything else they may be doing, to try out this particular innovation. Building the reflective healthcare organisation takes time. Therefore, those who are leading an initiative such as r-learning may have to pay particular attention to the issues of observability and relative advantage, mentioned earlier, if energy, commitment and interest are to be maintained.

Adopting an innovation: the case of an English primary care trust

In 2003, a large primary care trust in the UK embarked on a process of r-learning for all its clinical staff. The trust regarded this as an innovation and called it 'clinical reflection'. The goal was to improve the quality of services through better teamworking, and to do this by making learning through reflection an organisation-wide work habit for all the clinical staff. This included such disciplines as podiatry, continence services, district nursing, intermediate care, school nursing and palliative care. The process required staff to complete a questionnaire called STEPs (Ghaye 2005), which invited individuals to reflect upon the question 'What is it like working here, doing what you do, every day, with the people you work with?' Data from this 50-statement questionnaire illuminated the ten metrics, team by team, shown on p. 73. The results of this were discussed in a series of reflective team meetings. One outcome of these meetings was a positive action plan for service improvement through even better teamworking. A second questionnaire called SURE (Ghaye 2005) was also used by teams, which enabled them to better understand the impact of the services they were managing and delivering to their service users. Although a small amount of work on clinical reflection had taken place in the two years before 2003 (regarded by some in the trust as the 'trial period'), the innovation was formally regarded as 'being launched' upon the appointment of a full-time project manager in 2003. By September 2006, just over 320 staff were engaged in this work habit. This represented, with a few small exceptions, almost total coverage and uptake within the trust. The pattern of adoption is shown in Fig. 2.5, based upon a census of staff using this form of r-learning at every eighth month since its start in 2003.

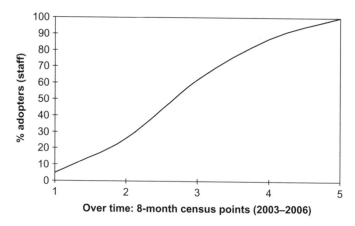

Figure 2.5 Percentage of adopters (staff) of clinical reflection over time within a primary care trust.

Coverage and uptake of r-learning

The coverage and uptake shown in Fig. 2.5 were greatly enhanced by the fact that the process of clinical reflection was:

- championed by the trust's executive nurse advisor and head of corporate services;
- being implemented by a dedicated project manager and a pool of trained facilitators (working in partnership with IRP-UK) for its duration;
- underpinned by appropriate financing mechanisms;
- monitored systematically with annual evaluations keeping achievements observable and known and informing future planning;
- kept visible across the organisation through regular presentations, to various staff groups, by the project manager and by articles in the trust's regular newsletter.

As far as this trust was able to, it got the politics and the support for this innovation right. The trust kept its focus on its staff teams and got the implementation right (see World Bank 2004). But this is not to say that the process was unproblematic.

The experiences of a district nursing team

Here is an example of the experiences of a district nursing team that adopted this particular innovation. It is interesting to see the way they put Rogers' (1983) requirements for a successful innovation in to their own words. Of special note is their way of reflecting on relative advantage, compatibility, complexity and observability.

Tarplee (2004) invited some district nurses to recall their experiences of clinical reflection, with regard to the point about relative advantage:

> We were positive and curious about what we were venturing into, and apprehensive about the constraints within a busy workload, what it involved and what the benefits would be to us as a team.

(Tarplee 2004, p. 4)

So who benefited from the process?

> We found the process to be focused, interesting, enjoyable and sometimes emotional. One of the questions we have asked ourselves is 'Who benefits from clinical reflection?' We believe that patients, the team, individuals and the PCT benefit.

(Tarplee 2004, p. 4)

What did staff learn when they reflected on the way they coped with their work pressures?

> When we discussed this within our reflective session, it was evident that there was diversity of opinion about work pressure. As a result, we devised an action plan which addressed specific areas. We changed our handover time to include all members of the team. We looked at the allocation of work in relation to workload dependency and the skill mix within the team. We also developed open communication within the team and with our clinical leader, which has led to different ways of working as natural changes occur.

(Tarplee 2004, p. 4).

And what did their patients think of their service?

> What was really interesting to us at the time was that, as part of the clinical reflection sessions, we asked a cross-section of patients – current and discharged patients – with different episodes of care what their real experience of care was.

(Tarplee 2004, p. 4)

How far did staff appear to their patients as though they were always in a hurry?

> In particular, we looked at time pressure – the extent to which people felt that staff always seemed to be in a hurry and under pressure. Our results demonstrated that none of our patients surveyed felt under pressure, or rushed. This told us that, even though we felt under pressure as a team, we were not portraying this message to our patients.

(Tarplee 2004, p. 4)

So what other things was the team of district nurses learning?

> This was a really positive message for us as a team. It gave us evidence that we were providing a professional and positive experience to our patients. We have

developed our own paperwork within the team to allow us to record the focus, action plans and outcomes of our reflective sessions. This also enables us to provide the evidence of how we spend our time in reflection and to show that we take action as a result of reflecting on our clinical practice.

(Tarplee 2004, p. 4)

Innovation as a non-linear dynamic system

Interestingly, if we change the way the same data are inputted for the r-learning innovation in the primary care trust mentioned above, a different picture emerges with regard to the adoption process. Figure 2.6 has been constructed using the actual (cumulative) number of staff adopting clinical reflection plotted against uptake census points every six months. The emerging adoption curve describes a much more valid uptake story – one that was essentially characterised by a 'rise and plateau' process with very active periods punctuated by periods of little activity. This can be accounted for by some facilitation difficulties, financial challenges, clinical team busyness and scheduling of teams to embrace the process, especially across the summer (holiday) months, for example. The work of Van de Ven *et al.* (1999) sheds more light on Fig. 2.6.

We should not underestimate the fact that when planning for innovation adoption, it is wise to pay attention to, and not downplay, the messy, often discontinuous nature of it, particularly when it is scaled up (Yin 1978). It does not always follow an S-curve. Nutley *et al.* (2002) suggest that adoption of an innovation may at first be related to the prospect

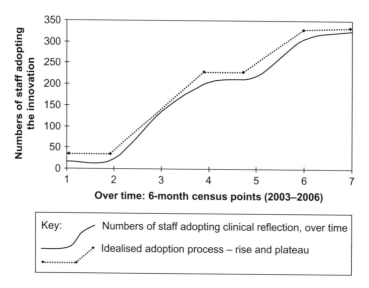

Figure 2.6 Numbers of adopters (staff) of clinical reflection over time within a primary care trust.

of new or better performance. Over time, others may adopt it in order to seek some kind legitimacy (DiMaggio & Powell 1983, O'Neill *et al.* 1998, Westphal *et al.* 1997). They say that this pattern of behaviour is heightened during times of high uncertainty, when organisations are more likely to imitate others, especially those perceived to be norm setters.

Innovation is not always orderly

In much of the literature on the adoption of innovation, an impression is created that this is a linear rather than a non-linear process (Radnor & Robinson 2000). Framing adoption in a linear way implies that the process is an orderly one. More recently, with innovation processes being researched more widely, the linear frame is increasingly giving way to a non-linear one (Calantone *et al.* 1988, Ettlie 1980, Josty 1990, King 1992, Kline 1985, Rickards 1996).

In the first part of this book, I referred to two metaphors that I would use to help describe the process of building a reflective healthcare organisation. Taken together they created the image of 'journeying over rough ground'. Nutley *et al.* (2002) suggest that more recent studies have characterised innovation as a journey that is neither sequential nor orderly but is messy and unpredictable. It is from the work of Van de Ven *et al.* (1999) that we get a real understanding of *innovation as a journey*. They describe its key characteristics thus:

- The innovation journey is about the many, not the few. It consists of the accretion of numerous events, performed by many people, over an extended period of time. Innovation is not about the action of an individual, on a particular date and time.
- The initiation of innovation is triggered by 'shocks', not simply by persuasion. One such 'shock' occurs when a threshold of dissatisfaction is reached with current circumstances. Gladwell (2005) would describe this as a tipping point where staff take action to resolve their current dissatisfaction.
- Innovation does not proceed in a simple linear sequence of stages and sub-stages. More realistically it splinters into complex bundles of innovative actions and divergent paths of activities by different organisational units. I return to this point below when describing action pathways-to-scale.
- Setbacks are frequently encountered during the innovation process because plans go awry or unanticipated organisational events change plans and alter what is possible. During times like these, the innovation might be suffering from 'rejection', might need to be adapted further or might be in gestation mode.
- Innovation receptiveness is enhanced if the innovation is developed in-house.
- Management cannot ensure innovation success but can influence its odds. The odds of success increase if those involved reflect on and

learn from their experiences of implementation (after Van de Ven *et al.* 1999, pp. 10–11).

The importance of change knowledge

Van de Ven *et al.* (1999) provide what Fullan (2005) calls 'change knowledge'; in other words, an understanding and insight about the processes of change and the key drivers that make for successful change in practice. 'The presence of change knowledge does not guarantee success, but its absence ensures failure' (Fullan 2005, p. 54). In reviewing 20 years of innovative processes that do and do not work, Fullan (2005) came up with eight drivers for effective and lasting change. They are:

- *Engaging people's moral purposes:* This is knowledge about the 'why' of change, the moral purposes of the innovation. Arguably in healthcare, this is centrally about committing to provide the best possible care for all patients.
- *Building capacity:* This is about the policies, strategies and resources that are required to enable staff to increase their collective power to move the system forward. It is also about creating a new shared identity and motivation to work together for greater change.
- *Understanding the change process:* This is understanding of the complexity and the energy and commitment required to be innovative. It also involves understanding the impact on staff of the 'implementation dip' (things getting worse before they get better).
- *Developing cultures for learning:* This is about establishing the organisational conditions for success. Central to this are forms of r-learning where staff learn from each other (the knowledge dimension) and become collectively committed to implementing the innovation (the affective dimension).
- *Developing cultures of evaluation:* This goes hand in hand with the previous driver. It is a way of sorting out promising practices from not-so-promising practices.
- *Focusing on leadership for change:* This involves knowing what kinds of leader and leadership are best suited for which kinds of innovation adoption process and how to produce leaders who have change knowledge.
- *Fostering coherence making:* If you believe that innovation is a non-linear, dynamic process, then effective and lasting change will occur only if there are staff in the organisation who can constantly keep the innovation process a coherent one. This means aligning values and actions, joining up the dots and relating the parts to the bigger picture.
- *Cultivating tri-level development:* This reminds us that in this book, when we talk about building a reflective healthcare organisation, we are talking about changing not individuals or teams but the whole organisation. This is why the scaling-up process can be called 'tri-level'. Fullan puts it thus:

We need to change individuals, but also to change contexts. We need to develop better individuals while we simultaneously develop better organisations and systems . . . For our purposes, we need only say, beware of the individualistic bias where the tacit assumption is that if we change enough individuals, then the system will change. In such cases, change won't happen. We need to change systems at the same time. To change individuals and systems simultaneously, we must provide more learning in context – that is learning in the actual situations we want to change.

(Fullan 2005, p. 58)

This change knowledge that Fullan talks about also needs to involve an appreciation that prior patterns of development and interaction both constrain and define opportunities for future innovation activities (Arthur 1994, Garcia-Pont & Nohria 2002, Gulati 1995, Walker *et al.* 1997). Staff, and therefore organisations, have memories.

The work of Greenhalgh *et al.* (2004) and a multidisciplinary view

Greenhalgh *et al.* (2004) asked: 'How can we spread and sustain innovations in health service delivery and organisation?' They defined innovation in service delivery and organisation as a novel set of behaviours, routines and ways of working that are directed at improving health outcomes, administrative efficiency, cost-effectiveness or users' experience and that are implemented by planned and coordinated actions. They distinguished among *diffusion* (passive spread), *dissemination* (active and planned efforts to persuade target groups to adopt an innovation), *implementation* (active and planned efforts to mainstream an innovation within an organisation), and *sustainability* (making an innovation routine until it reaches obsolescence).

Greenhalgh *et al.* took a systematic look at 13 research traditions relevant to the diffusion of innovation in health service organisations. I summarise the essence of these below. After this I add two more traditions to the list that are particularly relevant in the context of healthcare reforms today: appreciative inquiry and participative and appreciative action research (PA^{2}R). I describe the former in some detail in action step 3 of this book. I summarise Greenhalgh *et al.*'s (2004) research traditions in this way:

- *Rural sociology:* Rogers (1995) first developed the concept of the diffusion of innovations. He is best known for his S-curve, which describes this process.
- *Medical sociology:* Innovation theory is applied to doctors' clinical behaviour (e.g. Coleman *et al.* 1966) and forms the foundation for the development of network analysis, defined as the systematic study of 'who knows whom' and 'who copies whom' (Burt 1973).

- *Communication studies:* This studies the way in which new information is transmitted by the mass media or interpersonal communication. Research measures the speed and direction of the message's transmission and studies the impact of altering key variables such as the style of the message, the communication channel (spoken, written, etc.) and the nature of exposure (Rogers and Kincaid 1981).
- *Marketing:* This is essentially about efforts to increase the perceived benefits or reduce the perceived costs of an innovation in the eyes of potential adopters and the development of mathematical models to predict adoption behaviour (Bass 1969).
- *Development studies:* This tradition helps deepen our appreciation of the political, technological and ideological context of the innovation and any dissemination programme. Two important contributions from this tradition have been: (i) that the meaning of an innovation for the agency that introduces it may be very different from that held by the intended adopters, and (ii) that 'innovation–system fit' (related to the interaction between the innovation and its potential context) is generally a more valid and useful construct than 'innovation attributes' (often assumed to be fixed properties of the innovation in any context) (Bourdenave 1976).
- *Health promotion:* Here, innovations are defined as good ideas for healthy behaviours and lifestyles and include various models of partnership and community development (Potvin *et al.* 2001).
- *Evidence-based medicine:* This tradition is essentially about innovations defined as health technologies and practices supported by sound research evidence. Until recently, the spread of innovation in this tradition was seen as a linear and technical process, at the level of the individual, and hence was described as changes in clinicians' behaviour in line with evidence-based guidelines (Granados *et al.* 1997). This has given way to an understanding that individual change often requires changing the system (Grimshaw *et al.* 2004). What counts as sound research evidence is contested and must be continually interpreted and re-framed in accordance with the local context and priorities, a process that often involves power struggles among various professional groups (Ferlie *et al.* 2001).
- *Studies of the structural determinants of organisational innovativeness:* These are studies of the ways in which organisational innovativeness is regarded as being influenced primarily by structural determinates, especially size, functional differentiation (an internal division of labour), the amount of slack resources, and so on.
- *Studies of organisational process, context and culture:* This tradition focuses on an organisation's prevailing culture and climate, notably in relation to leadership style, power balances, social relations and attitudes towards risk-taking.
- *Inter-organisational studies:* Here, an organisation's innovativeness is 'situated' or related to the influence other organisations have upon it,

particularly inter-organisational communication, collaboration, competition and norm setting. Networking (Granovetter & Soong 1983) and inter-organisational norms, fads and fashions are seen as a key mechanism for spreading ideas among organisations (Abrahamson 1991, Abrahamson & Fairchild 1999).

- *Knowledge-based approaches to innovation in organisations:* Here, innovation and diffusion are radically re-defined as the construction and distributed of knowledge (Nonaka & Takeuchi 1995). A critical new concept is the organisation's absorptive capacity for new knowledge (Zahra & George 2002).
- *Narrative organisational studies:* In this field, an innovative organisation is one in which new stories can be told and one that has the capacity to capture and circulate these stories (Czarniawska 1998, Gabriel 2000).
- *Complexity studies:* This tradition is derived from general systems theory and regards innovation as complex responses of humans, relating to one another, in local situations. The diffusion of innovations is seen as a highly organic and adaptive process in which the organisation adapts to the innovation and the innovation is adapted to the organisation (Fonseca 2001). Later I say more about the importance of being an adaptive organisation and how this is a significant characteristic of the reflective healthcare organisation.

To this list of 13 I add two more items:

- *Appreciative inquiry:* This emerging tradition is based upon the four ideas that the world is socially constructed, that these constructions inform action, that realities are produced in relationships, and that meaning is created through appreciation. This is appreciation in three senses: 'First, as a deep awareness of the complex potential for interpreting the nature and value of words or actions. Second, as the affirming of meaning and value of words and actions. Third, as adding to the meaning and value of words and actions' (Anderson *et al.* 2006, p. 11). This appreciative approach allows views and values to circulate more freely within the organisation. At the intersection of multiple realities we find creative growth points. The diffusion of innovation is about getting to the root causes of success and growing in this direction. Diffusion is not about fixing the problems, freeing up the bottlenecks, managing resistance and simply leaving the successful aspects of the innovation to look after themselves.
- *Participative and appreciative action research (PA²R):* This has emerged from the broad action research tradition, which has many forms, such as participative and collaborative action research, emancipatory action research and action sciences. Action research consists of a family of methodologies that pursue outcomes of both action (improvement) and research (understanding). It uses a process of inquiry that alternates between action and systematic reflection, works with (not on) people, and does not separate theory from practice. PA²R is a recent

style of research that emphasises the power of asking the positive question and is a strength-based rather than deficit-based approach to improving the work and working life of individuals and groups/ teams within organisations. For further details of PA²R see Melander-Wikman *et al.* (2006) and Bergmark *et al.* (2007).

References

Abrahamson, E. (1991) Managerial fads and fashions: the diffusion and rejection of innovation. *California Management Review* **16**, 586–612.

Abrahamson, E. (1996) Management fashion. *Academy of Management Review* **21**(1), 254–85.

Abrahamson, E. & Fairchild, G. (1999) Management fashion: lifecycles, triggers and collective learning processes. *Administrative Sciences Quarterly* **44**(4), 708–40.

Amabile, T. (1998) How to kill creativity. *Harvard Business Review* **76**, 76–87.

Amar, A.D. (2001) Leading for innovation through symbiosis. *European Journal of Innovation Management* **4**(3), 126–32.

Anderson, H., Cooperrider, D., Gergen, K.J. *et al.* (2006) *The Appreciative Organization.* Taos Institute Publications, Chagrin Falls, OH.

Arthur, W.B. (1994) *Increasing Returns and Path Dependence in the Economy.* University of Michigan Press, Ann Arbor, MI.

Axtell, C.M., Holman, D.J., Unsworth, K.L., *et al.* (2000) Shopfloor innovation: facilitating the suggestion and implementation of ideas. *Journal of Occupational and Organizational Psychology* **73**, 265–85.

Baer, M. & Frese, M. (2003) Innovation is not enough: climates for initiative and psychological safety, process innovations and firm performance. *Journal of Organizational Behaviour* **24**, 45–68.

Bass, F.M. (1969) A new product growth model for consumer durables. *Management Science* **13**(5), 215–27.

Benkhoff, B. (1997) Disentangling organisational commitment: the dangers of OCQ for research and policy. *Personnel Review* **26**(1/2), 114–31.

Bergmark, U., Ghaye, T. & Alerby, E. (2007) Reflective and appreciative actions that support the building of ethical places and spaces. *Reflective Practice* **8**(3), Forthcoming.

Berwick, D.M. (2003) Disseminating innovations in health care. *JAMA* **289**(15), 1969–75.

Bourdenave, J.D. (1976) Communication of agricultural innovations in Latin America: the need for new models. *Communication Research* **3**(2), 135–54.

Burt, R.S. (1973) The differential impact of social integration on participation in the diffusion of innovations. *Social Science Research* **2**(2), 125–44.

Calantone, R.J., Di Benedetto, A. & Meloche, M. (1988) Strategies of product and process innovation: a loglinear analysis. *R & D Management* **18**, 13–21.

Charters, W.W. & Pellegrin, R.S. (1972) Barriers to the innovation process: four case studies of differentiated staffing. *Educational Agricultural Quarterly* (9), 3–4.

Coleman, J.S., Katz, E. & Menzel, H. (1966) *Medical Innovations: A Diffusion Study.* Bobbs-Merrill, New York.

Cooper, R.B. and Zmud, R.W. (1990) Information technology implementation research: a technology diffusion approach. *Management Science* **36**(2), 123–39.

Czarniawska, B. (1998) *A Narrative Approach to Organisation Studies.* Sage, London.

Department of Health (2000) An organisation with a memory. Report of an expert group on learning from adverse events in the NHS chaired by the Chief Medical Officer. Department of Health, London.

DiMaggio, P. & Powell, W. (1983) The iron cage revisited: institutional isomorphism and collective rationality in organisation fields. *American Sociological Review* **48**, 147–60.

Ettlie, J.E. (1980) Manpower flows and the innovation process. *Management Science* **26**, 1086–95.

Ferlie, E., Gabbay, J., FitzGerald, L., *et al.* (2001) Evidence-based medicine and organisational change: an overview of some recent qualitative research. In *Organisational Behaviour and Organisational Studies in Health Care: Reflections on the Future* (ed. L. Ashburner). Palgrave, Basingstoke.

Fernández, A.M. (2001) Innovation processes in an emergency department. *European Journal of Innovation Management* **4**(4), 168–78.

Fonseca, J. (2001) *Complexity and Innovation in Organisations.* Routledge, London.

Fullan, M. (2005). *Leadership and Sustainability: System Thinkers in Action.* Corwin, Thousand Oaks, CA.

Gabriel, Y. (2000) *Storytelling in Organisations: Facts, Fictions and Fantasies.* Oxford University Press, Oxford.

Garcia-Pont, C. & Nohria, N. (2002) Local versus global mimetism: the dynamics of alliance formation in the automobile industry. *Strategic Management Journal* **23**, 307–21.

Ghaye (2005) *Developing the Reflective Healthcare Team.* Blackwell Publishing, Oxford.

Gladwell, M. (2005) *The Tipping Point: How Little Things Can Make A Big Difference.* Abacus, London.

Granados, A., Jonsson, E., Banta, H.D., *et al.* (1997) EUR-ASSESS project subgroup report on dissemination and impact. *International Journal of Technology Assessment in Health Care* **13**(2), 220–86.

Granovetter, M. & Soong, R. (1983) Threshold models of diffusion and collective behaviour. *Journal of Mathematical Sociology* **9**, 165–79.

Greenhalgh, T., Robert, G., MacFarlane, F., *et al.* (2004) Diffusion of innovations in service organisations: systematic review and recommendations. *Milbank Quarterly* **82**(4), 581–629.

Grimshaw, J.M., Thomas, R.E., MacLennan, G., *et al.* (2004) Effectiveness and efficiency of guideline dissemination and implementation strategies. *Health Technology Assessment Report* **8**(6), 1–72.

Gulati, R. (1995) Social structure and alliance formation patterns: a longitudinal analysis. *Administrative Science Quarterly* **40**, 619–52.

Halladay, M. & Bero, L. (2000) Implementing evidence-based practice in health care. *Public Money and Management* **20**(4), 43–50.

Hellström, T., Jacob, M. & Malmquist, U. (2002) Guiding innovation socially and cognitively: the innovation team model at Skanova Networks. *European Journal of Innovation Management* **5**(3), 172–80.

Institute for Healthcare Improvement (2003) *The Breakthrough Series: IHI's Collaborative Model for Achieving Breakthrough Improvement.* Institute for Healthcare Improvement, Boston, MA.

Institute of Medicine (1999) To err is human: building a safer health system. Report brief. Available at http://newton.nap.edu/html/to_err_is_human/reportbrief.pdf

Institute of Reflective Practice UK (2007) *STEPs.* IRP-UK Publications, Gloucester.

Johannessen, J.A., Olsen B. & Lumpkin, G. (2001) Innovation as newness: what is new, how new, and new to whom? *European Journal of Innovation Management* **4**(1), 20–31.

Josty, P.L. (1990) A tentative model of the innovation process. *R & D Management* **20**, 35–45.

Kandampully, J. (2002) Innovation as the core competency of a service organisation: the role of technology, knowledge and networks. *European Journal of Innovation Management* **5**(1), 18–26.

Kegan, R. & Lahey, L. (2001) *Seven Languages for Transformation: How the Way We Talk Can Change the Way We Work.* Jossey-Bass, San Francisco, CA.

King, N. (1992) Modelling the innovation process: an empirical comparison of approaches. *Journal of Occupational and Organizational Psychology* **65**, 89–101.

King, N. & Anderson, N. (1995) Innovation in working groups. In *Innovation and Creativity at Work* (eds M.A. West & J.L. Farr). John Wiley & Sons, Chichester.

Kitson, A., Harvey, G. & McCormack, B. (1998) Enabling the implementation of evidence based practice: a conceptual framework. *Quality in Health Care* **7**, 149–51.

Kline, S.J. (1985) Innovation is not a linear process. *Research Management* **28**, 36–45.

Lideway, E.C. (2004) Designing the workplace for learning and innovation. *Development and Learning in Organizations* **18**(5), 10–13.

Lyall, J. (2006) At risk: the safety agency that failed to set the world on fire. *Health Service Journal*, 28 September, 14–15.

McAdam, R. & McClelland, J. (2002) Individual and team-based idea generation within innovation management: organisational and research agendas. *European Journal of Management* **5**(2), 86–97.

Melander-Wikman, A., Jansson, M. & Ghaye, T. (2006) Reflections on an appreciative approach to empowering elderly people, in home healthcare. *Reflective Practice* **7**(4), 423–44.

Miller, D. (1990) *The Icarus Paradox*. HarperCollins, New York.

Mohrle, M. & Pannenbacker, T. (1997) Problem-driven inventing: a concept for strong solutions to inventive tasks. *Creativity and Innovation Management* **6**(4), 234–48.

National Audit Office (2006) *A Safer Place for Patients: Learning to Improve Patient Safety*. The Stationery Office, London.

Nonaka, I. & Takeuchi, H. (1995) *The Knowledge Creation Company: How Japanese Companies Create the Dynamics of Innovation*. Oxford University Press, New York.

Nutley, S., Walter, I. & Davies, H. (2002) Conceptual synthesis 1: learning from the diffusion of innovations. Working paper 10. ESRC UK Centre for Evidence Based Policy and Research, London.

Olin, T. & Wickenberg, J. (2001) Rule breaking in new product development: crime or necessity? *Creativity and Innovation Management* **10**(1), 15–25.

O'Neill, H.M., Pouder, R.W. & Buchholtz, A.K. (1998) Patterns in the diffusion of strategies across organisations; insights from the innovation diffusion literature. *Academy of Management Review* **23**(1), 98–114.

Osborne, S.P. (1998) *Voluntary Organizations and Innovation in Public Services*. Routledge, London.

Peters, T.J. & Waterman, R.H. (1982) *In Search of Excellence: Lessons from America's Best Run Companies*. Harper & Row, New York.

Pokhrel, S. (2006) Scaling up health interventions in resource-poor countries: what role does research in stated-preference framework play? *Health Research Policy and Systems* **4**, 4.

Potvin, L., Haddad, S. & Frohlich, K.L. (2001) Beyond process and outcome evaluation: a comprehensive approach for evaluating health promotion programmes. *WHO Regional Publications: European Series* **92**, 45–62.

Radnor, Z. & Robinson, J. (2000) Benchmarking innovation: a short report. *Journal of Creativity and Innovation Management* **9**(1), 3–13.

Rickards, T. (1996) The management of innovation: recasting the role of creativity. *European Journal of Work and Organizational Psychology* **5**(1), 13–27.

Rogers, E.M. (1983) *Diffusion of Innovations*, 3rd edn. Free Press, New York.

Rogers, E.M. (1995) *Diffusion of Innovations*, 4th edn. Free Press, New York.

Rogers, E.M. & Kincaid, D.L. (1981) *Communication Networks: Toward a New Paradigm for Research*. Free Press, New York.

Rogers, E.M. & Scott, K. (1997) The diffusion of innovations model and outreach from the National Network of Libraries of Medicine to Native American communities. Draft paper prepared for the National Network of Libraries of Medicine, Pacific Northwest Region, Seattle, WA. Available at http://nnlm.gov/evaluation/pub/rogers/

Sanson-Fisher, R.W. (2004) Diffusion of innovation theory for clinical change. *Medical Journal of Australia* **180**, S55–56.

Shalley, C.E., Gilson, L.L. & Blum, T.C. (2000) Matching creativity requirements and the work environment: effects on satisfaction and intentions to leave. *Academy of Management Journal* **43**(2), 215–23.

Slappendel, C. (1996) Perspectives on innovation in organizations. *Organization Studies* **17**(1), 107–29.

Suliman, A.M.T. (2001) Are we ready to innovate? Work climate-readiness to innovate relationship: the case of Jordan. *Creativity and Innovation Management* **10**(1), 49–59.

Tarplee, M. (2004) Clinical reflection . . . what's been happening? *In Touch* **13**, 4–5. Available at www.easternbirminghampct.nhs.uk/docs/intouch/In%20Touch%20-%20Issue%2013.pdf

Van de Ven, A.H., Polley, D., Garud, R. & Venkataraman. S. (1999) *The Innovation Journey*. Oxford University Press, New York and Oxford.

Walker, G., Kogut, B. & Shan, W. (1997) Social capital, structural holes and the formation of an industry network. *Organisation Science* **8**, 2.

Walshe, K. & Rundall, T.G. (2001) Evidence-base management: from theory to practice in health care. *Milbank Quarterly* **79**(3), 429–57.

Weaver, M. (2006) Britons most obese in Europe. Guardian Unlimited, 10 October. Available at http://society.guardian.co.uk/health/story/0,,1892098,00.htm

West, M. (1990) The social psychology of innovation in groups. In *Innovation and Creativity at Work* (eds M.A. West & J.L. Farr). John Wiley & Sons, Chichester.

Westphal, J.D., Gulati, R. & Shortell, S.M. (1997) Customization or conformity? An institutional and network perspective on the content and consequences of TQM adoption. *Administrative Science Quarterly* **42**(2), 366–94.

Wheatley, M.J. (2002) *Turning to One Another: Simple Conversations to Restore Hope to the Future*. Berrett-Koehler, San Francisco, CA.

Wolfe, R.A. (1994) Organisational innovation: review, critique and suggested research directions. *Journal of Management Studies* **31**(3), 405–31.

World Bank (2004) Lessons: scaling up successful efforts to reduce poverty. Available at: http://info.worldbank.org/etools/reducingpoverty/docs/shanghailessons.pdf#search=%22lessons%3A%20scaling%20up%20successful%20efforts%22

World Health Organization (2004) An approach to rapid scale-up: using HIV/AIDS treatment and care as an example. HIV/Aids, Tuberculosis and Malaria Evidence and Information for Policy. World Health Organization, Geneva.

Yin, R.K. (1978) Organizational innovation: a psychologist's view. In *The Diffusion of Innovations: An Assessment* (eds M. Radnor, I. Feller & E. Rogers). Northwestern University, Center for the Interdisciplinary Study of Science and Technology, Evanston, IL.

Zahra, A.S. & George, G. (2002) Absorptive capacity: a review, reconceptualisation and extension. *Academy of Management Review* **27**(2), 185–203.

Chapter 3

Action step 3: journeying along action pathways-to-scale

In this third step over the 'rough ground' I want to set out some more ways to make progress towards building a reflective healthcare organisation. Collectively I refer to these as action *pathways-to-scale*. Six are described and illustrated. I talk about the promise each action pathway holds. Action step 3 contains six major ideas bundles. They are:

Bundle 1 **Values**
In this part of the book I identify a number of action pathways-to-scale. There are no right or wrong pathways to follow – only what is right for your organisation given your assessment of its starting position. Each pathway describes a journey across 'rough ground'. I begin with the values pathway because values affect what we feel and think. Therefore, they affect the quality of our practice. They provide the reasons for our actions. Some of the rough ground involves understanding that what we say is not always what we do.

Bundle 2 **Conversation**
This bundle contains a call to change the way we normally view our work and interactions with others. I suggest that conversations about problems end up being a problem because problems tend to suck all the energy out of us, as we try to 'fix' or get rid of them. As an alternative, I make a case for focusing on successes, to use our energy to find the root causes of them, and then to work out ways to experience success more frequently. This involves using the power of the positive question and understanding how we can 'tip' conversations away from problems and towards a more sustained consideration of successes.

Bundle 3 **User**
This bundle intersects with the previous two around the idea of 'the value of being valued'. It describes, and gives reasons for, building a language of positive regard with service users. Trust, open and reflective listening, positive engagement and appropriate feedback are important components of such a language. Some of the rough ground within this bundle of ideas may well concern responses to the questions 'What can I learn from service users' experience?' and 'How can learning from service users become an organisation-wide, reflective work habit?'

Bundle 4 **Leadership**
Holding centre stage within this bundle are two ideas about leadership. They are *leading through appreciation* and *tipping-point leadership*. I argue

that scaling up r-learning through this action pathway requires leadership that can re-frame personally constructed realities, appreciate the positive and see how the future unfolds from the present. I align these with the intentions of r-learning described in Fig. 0.2.

Bundle 5   Team

Some of the potential rough ground in this bundle of ideas may well be associated with my argument that scaling up r-learning is not simply a matter of creating more and more reflective teams. Then, as if by some kind of magic, this leads to something we might call the reflective health-care organisation. Getting a 'critical mass' of reflective teams inside the organisation is only one part, albeit an important part, of the process. Two other important parts are increasing the frequency of what I refer to as 'have moments', additionally exploring ways to nurture collective wisdom.

Bundle 6   Network

The central idea within this final bundle is the notion of the networked organisation. I set out the essential characteristics of a network and apply the ideas of nodes (people) and links (interactions) to healthcare. Progress along this pathway entails encountering the complementary processes of the *appreciative sharing of knowledge* and the *mapping of knowledge-sharing networks*. The bundle concludes by suggesting how these twin processes can be key enablers to scaling up r-learning.

To help you navigate your way through action step 3, these ideas are linked together into a mind map (Fig. 3.1).

What is a pathway-to-scale?

Thus far in this book, I have referred to the necessity to identify and make progress along action pathways-to-scale. I have identified six pos-sible and potentially useful pathways (see Table 0.3). In the introduction, I talked about successful action being about choosing and following the most appropriate path. Successful action here means scaling up r-learning so that it becomes a collegial and useful organisation-wide work habit. Each action pathway enables us to make progress towards building a reflective healthcare organisation. There is no right or wrong pathway. Each pathway brings with it its own promise. Neither is there a predeter-mined and universally agreed sequence of pathways to follow. There is only what is right for your organisation, given your assessment of where it is, organisationally, and what its priorities are. The key question is: What is or are the most appropriate path(s) to follow that might enable you to scale up reflective learning, thus moving it from an individualistic pursuit to a collective and productive work habit? I wish to argue that progress along a values pathway is fundamental, so I discuss this in more detail than other pathways-to-scale.

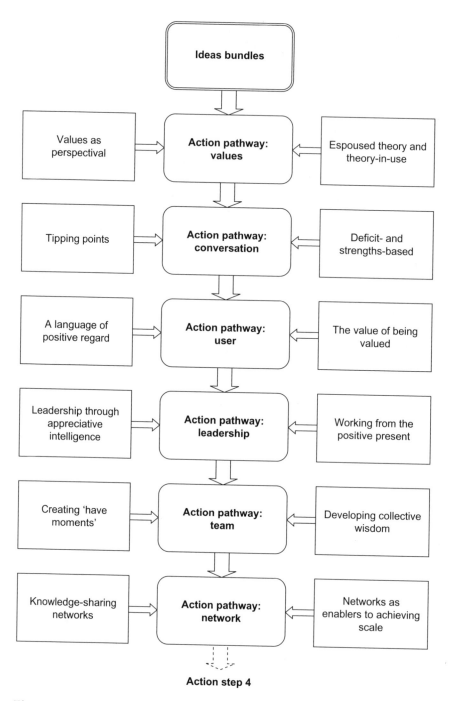

Figure 3.1 Mind map for action step 3: journeying along action pathways-to-scale.

Action pathway: values

The action here is essentially about working towards becoming a reflective organisation by building an understanding of, and congruence between, espoused values and values-in-action. So what are values? What are they about? Do you and your colleagues have them? Do you know where to look for them? How far do you share the same values with others? How far do they influence what you do? Or, put another way, how far does knowing your values help you in your work?

Values are everywhere, but we need to wear certain reflective lenses to fully appreciate them. Values help us achieve the vision we have of a good-quality healthcare service. This is why they are an important action pathway. Values provide a key means through which a vision becomes part of the everyday working life of staff and experiences of service users. Values need to be articulated, lived and acknowledged by all those developing, managing, evaluating and using healthcare services. It should be possible to track an organisation's values through all aspects of healthcare, wherever this may be – in leadership and management, finance and estates, clinical services, teaching and learning, in external relations and customer care, in acute and community settings, and so on. Crucially, we need to reflect upon the extent to which our espoused values (what we say) match are values-in-action.

How values manifest themselves

Values manifest themselves in things we read, such as in a mission statement and in business and action plans. Sometimes we need go no further than the title of major government policy documents to get the feel for the values that might be espoused therein; good examples of which are *Working Together – Learning Together* (Department of Health 2001), *Liberating the Talents* (Department of Health 2002a), *Shifting the Balance of Power* (Department of Health 2002b) and *Improving Working Lives* (Department of Health 2002c). There are many values embedded in the Nursing and Midwifery Council's (2002) statement *Supporting Nurses and Midwives through Lifelong Learning*. These are values related to the nature of staff support and commitments to lifelong learning. When reading the Commission for Health Improvement's (2003) report on the NHS, *Getting Better?*, we read about what is valued by the Commission, namely the experience of those who use the NHS. The Commission also leads us into the complex area of value judgements. Interestingly, halfway through the ten-year NHS Plan in the UK, developing a patient-led NHS has shifted everyone's focus on to the crucial area of commissioning. Expert, imaginative commissioning is central to a patient-led NHS, as are changes to the organisation of primary care, in order to make the NHS fit for the twenty-first century. In a letter to all trusts about strengthening commissioning, Sir Ian Carruthers, the acting NHS chief executive, in May 2006, refers to a vision entitled 'Health Reform in England: Update and Next Steps'. In this is an outline for taking forward the reform of the NHS. The framework is full of *reform values*, such as:

- more choice and a much stronger voice for patients (demand-side reforms);
- money following the patients, rewarding the best and most efficient providers, and giving others the incentive to improve (transactional reforms);
- more diverse providers, with more freedom to innovate and improve services (supply-side reforms);
- a framework of system management, regulation and decision-making that guarantees safety and quality, fairness, equity and value for money.

Should staff be rewarded for being nice to patients?

Values matter. Values are not fluffy or abstract things but essential and concrete. It is important to remember that in our daily interaction with patients and clients, we promote, or put into action, values all of the time. Many of us are not aware that we are doing this. R-learning helps to heighten our awareness of our personal and shared values and how far we put them into practice. In order to be professional and act ethically, we need to learn how to be explicit about the values we hold and which values are the most important to us. These are what we can call *core values*. A lack of explicitness makes it harder to have a shared vision about the kinds and quality of service we want for service users. Through reflective conversations, we may come to agree a number of core values. These then become *your* values rather than those imposed on you from elsewhere and outside of your organisation.

The *Nursing Times* printed an article called 'A motivational scheme at a London hospital encourages nurses to be helpful and friendly to patients' (O'Dowd 2006), full of values about the way staff should (or were being encouraged or supported) to interact with patients and why. Below is an excerpt from the article. What values can you spot?

> One of the obvious assumptions about nurses is that they will be nice to patients. Of course the vast majority are but this attitude can sometimes be taken for granted. This is why a motivational scheme was set up on general medical wards at King's College Hospital NHS Trust in London, six months ago, and is about to be rolled out to other departments in the trust including surgery, specialist medicine and A & E. The FISH scheme – inspired by a programme first used at a fish market in Seattle to boost sales – rewards staff seen being particularly nice or helpful to patients. It was introduced to King's after Selina Truman, head of nursing in general medicine at the trust, heard from a U.S. nurse about the approach to changing culture and improving ways of working.

The technique comprises four elements:

Making my day – doing something to make someone else's day better;

Being present – engaging with the person you are with;

–Being playful – having fun during work;

Choosing a great attitude – having a positive attitude while at work.

Under the scheme, staff who are observed by sisters and matrons putting the FISH philosophy into practice are given a thank-you card in recognition of their attitude . . . Every two weeks, these cards are put into a draw and the winner gets a voucher for a free coffee and cookie in the staff café . . .

Angela Pennock, a matron in King's general medical care group, said that more than 1,000 thank-you cards had been issued to staff. 'At first, staff were a bit suspicious because they wondered how it was going to work and what it was for. But we explained when we launched it that we wanted to make work more enjoyable,' she said. 'So often, the public thinks that nurses are angels and that it is a vocation. There is a worry that the good attitude of nurses is taken for granted. This was something about employers recognising the work that nurses do and valuing the input that they give' she added.

(O'Dowd 2006, p. 9)

Some important questions

- What values are embedded in this article?
- Why do you think such a scheme is necessary?
- How far do nurses need inducements to be nice to patients?
- What are the root causes of nurses not being able to spend quality time with their patients and caring for them in an appropriate manner?
- How far is importing a scheme from the fishing industry a good idea?

Carr (1992) says that values are of 'quite considerable importance' and:

. . . unlike other sorts of preferences which are based merely on personal taste or natural disposition, values are standardly a consequence of something approaching intelligent deliberation and are thus, in principle, susceptible of rational appraisal and re-appraisal.

(Carr 1992, p. 244)

For example, you may have a view with regard to the UK government's establishment of foundation trusts. This view is unlikely to be based upon a whim or fancy but concerned more with a principled preference. By implication, this makes us valuing beings and our work value-laden.

In Ghaye (2005) I set out three important areas for r-learning with regard to values. They were about the nature and processes of:

- *Values clarification:*
  - Over what things do you and service users agree?
  - Why do you agree over these things?

- *Value conflicts:*
    - Over what things do you and service users disagree?
    - Why do you disagree over these things?
- *Value consensus:*
    - What does 'a quality service' mean to different stakeholders?
    - What rights and obligations do different stakeholders have?

In this next example we can find a consideration of each of these. It is part of an extract from an editorial by Sensky (2002) called 'Withdrawal of life sustaining treatment'.

When patients' autonomy and values conflict with the responsibilities of clinicians

Ms B, as she was called in court and in the media, was a 43 year old professional woman who in 1999 had a haemorrhage in a cavernous haemangioma in her upper spinal cord. After an almost complete recovery she had a re-bleed in February 2001, which rendered her quadriplegic and dependent on artificial ventilation. Specialists who reviewed her all agreed that she had a negligible chance of substantial recovery, and she was advised to consider specialist rehabilitation. Ms B went to great lengths to gather information about her prognosis. She remained adamant that living on a ventilator would be intolerable to her because of the level of dependence on others and the lack of control over her own body she would have, and she requested to have her ventilation discontinued. The clinicians treating her felt unable to carry out her wishes, and Ms B eventually took to court the NHS Trust treating her.

Dame Elizabeth Butler-Sloss judged that Ms B was indeed competent to decide on her treatment, and therefore her decisions about her treatment, whatever they were, must be respected. The judgment reviewed precedents for this, including the judge's own previous statement that 'a mentally competent patient has an absolute right to refuse to consent to treatment for any reason, rational or irrational, or for no reason at all, even where that decision may lead to his or her own death'.

(Sensky 2002, p. 175)

So what kinds of value position are being articulated here? What needs to be clarified further? What are the conflicts and the areas of consensus? Where do you stand in relation to each of the following questions?

- How far do you feel that the clinicians involved might begin to doubt their own competence when a patient makes a serious decision that goes against their professional advice?
- How far do you agree that any judgement about this case is dependent upon understanding how far Ms B. is capable of assimilating and

understanding information about her condition, appreciates the personal relevance of this information, is capable of discussing it with others, and is able to form judgements by weighing up the information she has acquired?

- How far do you feel that Ms B. is basing her decision upon her values? How far do you feel she values the continuing life she faced, particularly being dependent on others, as worse than death?
- How far do you feel that healthcare professionals must recognise the differences between personal values and professional knowledge?
- How far do you agree that values can, and often do, alter with changing health circumstances and experience?
- How far do you feel that what matters most here are Ms B.'s values at the time the decision needs to be made?

Values are perspectival

Values don't just come out of thin air. They come from the religious, spiritual, moral, ethical, professional and other beliefs we hold. They also come from the assumptions we make about ourselves and each other and what managing, delivering and using healthcare services is about. In this sense we can describe values as *perspectival*. This means that they reflect something about the particular and shared perspectives we have. Different individuals and groups of service users may hold different perspectives (or views) about what a healthcare professional does and stands for. These shape their understanding and expectations of, as well as their interactions with, professionals and services. The different perspectives an individual or group of healthcare professionals may have, with regard to the knowledge and skills needed for competent practice, might be informed by any one or more of the following (and other) perspectives:

- *Learning as a lifelong process:* critical curiosity, making connections, challenge, making meaning, staying up-to-date.
- *Spirituality:* developing self-awareness, awareness of others, awareness of the world around us and, for some, an awareness of a god or adherence to the words of scriptures.
- *Social development:* cooperation, teamworking, empathising.
- *Cultural awareness:* valuing difference and diversity positively.
- *Personal development:* self-esteem, self-efficacy, motivation for learning, emotional literacy.
- *Ethics:* what is right, socially just, honesty, fairness.

Different and shared perspectives

We all have different and shared perspectives on issues that we feel are important to us. Healthcare is one such issue. For example, Branthwaite (2005) aired some of the debates associated with euthanasia and physician-assisted suicide and, more specifically, about the moral and legal validity

of providing assistance to die. This debate has been fuelled by the publication of the report of a House of Lords select committee set up to consider
the Assisted Dying for the Terminally Ill Bill and the final determination
by the US courts that hydration and nutrition could lawfully be with-
drawn from a patient in a persistent vegetative state. What are some of the
principles and practicalities involved? Much will depend upon the perspectives of euthanasia and assisted death that you hold. How does this
issue make you feel about the principle of respect for personal autonomy?
How far do you feel that competent adults are entitled to withhold or
withdraw consent to their life-sustaining treatment? What do you feel
about the perspective that, although the motive may be benevolent, the
intention is to kill or to permit a preventable death? How do a patient's
dignity and quality of life shape your perspective? Responses to each of
these questions involve the making of value judgements.

In general, there are at least six other perspectives on values that are
worth acknowledging. They are not mutually exclusive. They are perspectives that can create value:

- blindness
- confusion
- tokenism
- conquest
- alienation
- conflict.

Value blindness

We know we have reasons for doing what we do, although we may not
always be fully aware of them. We may not call these reasons values, but
it is our values that indeed influence what and how well we do things.
Building the reflective healthcare organisation brings with it a need to
make that which is personally known (Polanyi 1958) more explicit and
publicly available for discussion and exploration. There are a range of
methods that help make the tacit more explicit. Some are paper-and-pencil
activities, and some more expressive (Ghaye & Lillyman 2001, Higgs &
Titchen 2001, Hunt & Sampson 1998, Kember *et al.* 2001, Novak 1998,
Parkinson 1997). Making the tacit more explicit might include the use of
painting, dance, music, photography, drama, mod-roc modelling, and so
on. Blindness can be addressed if we organise and sustain organisational
dialogues about values. It can also be addressed if a trust explicitly states
its values in its mission statement, trust profile, annual report and any
appropriate marketing and publicity materials that go outside the trust
or are placed strategically for users of services to read. We can find an
explicit (noticeable and visible) statement of values in one of the UK
NHS trusts that was awarded, in July 2005, the highest rating of three
stars in the Healthcare Commission's annual performance ratings. The
trust also won the *Health Service Journal*'s 'Acute Healthcare Organisation

of the Year' and 'Employer of the Year' awards. The trust serves a population of 150000 people through 4 hospitals, 5 health centres and 17 community clinics. Its values are:

- We will treat you politely and with honesty and respect.
- We will treat you fairly, based on your needs.
- We will involve you in decisions about your care and treatment
  and give you information which will allow you to make informed
  choices.
- We will, with your permission, keep a relative or named friend
  informed of your condition.
- We will respect your rights to privacy, dignity and confidentiality and
  keep your health and social care records secure. You can apply for
  access to see your records.
- We will give you information in an appropriate format and language,
  to suit your needs.
- We will provide extra help, if needed, for example, having someone
  to speak for you if necessary.

What is interesting is that in the current (at the time of writing) clinical
governance report of this trust, there is an explicit reference to the important role of what they call 'reflective discussions' with colleagues and
managers, around policies, procedures and guidelines. Included in this is
open communication with the public about services in the spirit of
improving relationships and understanding, joint working and continuing to strengthen its partnership arrangements with all stakeholders. The
challenge of making values more visible and known should not be
underestimated. Goldhammer (1966) reminds us:

> The vast majority ... of values and assumptions from which our ... profes-
> sional behaviour is governed are implicit. They're inarticulate, they're nebu-
> lous, they're buried someplace in our guts and they're not always very
> accessible ... We can't always rationalise exactly what we're doing ... We can't
> always make explicit the justifications for the acts we perpetrate ... Only after
> these things have been made explicit, have been brought to the point where
> you can enunciate the damn things, can we begin to value those that seem to
> have some ... integrity and disregard those that seem to be inane.

(Goldhammer 1966, p. 49)

Value confusion

This often arises from having a long list of values. Sometimes 'the more
the merrier' is a recipe for confusion. A list emerges and consensus rules.
There is nothing wrong with consensus, as long as it is a genuine consensus and not one that is forced upon staff due to time constraints or other
pressures from 'the top' or from outside. Sometimes it may be hard to

know what is and is not a value: 'Isn't everything we care about a value?' Some of the contents on these lists may by represented by a single word. Other parts of the list might contain lengthy phrases and statements of 'good intent'. It is wise to make time for conversations about clarifying confusion. Values need to be given a chance to bubble to the surface. A positive example of a short, unambiguous values statement is drawn from another of the 2005 three-star, award-winning NHS trusts. They put things like this.

Our values:

- We put our patients first.
- We treat everyone with respect and dignity.
- We work purposefully and responsibly.
- We are dedicated to continuous improvement.
- We work in effective and efficient partnerships and teams.

Value confusion, obscurity and lack of clarity fog decision-making. Value confusion needs to be addressed systematically through appropriately scheduled, and inclusive, reflective conversations.

Value tokenism

This occurs within organisations, and especially within some teams, that are able, at that time, to make no more than a token effort or gesture in the direction of addressing the centrality of values in their practice. Another expression of tokenism is about making statements that we claim to be team values, actually writing them down, and then thinking 'Tick the box – job done!' This tokenism may be fleeting or a more subtle or sustained act of avoidance of the implications for our sense of identity and self-worth. Tokenism can happen for a variety of reasons. Sometimes it happens when a team sees the process of values clarification as just another task and something that teams have to do. It takes courage to live by the values we say we believe in. It takes personal and collective effort to put our values into action. A big effort is needed for everyone to get to know what the trust, team and individual values are. Values mean something only when they are put into practice. Espousing certain values is an important step, but it is not simply what we say that counts in healthcare: what we do counts more.

This is communicated vividly by another of the award-winning NHS trusts in 2005. The trust's aspiration is to be the best hospital in the NHS in the UK. The trust believes that this vision will be realised by planning, organising and delivering services to achieve three things: (i) the best possible care for patients, (ii) improved health for the community and (iii) joy and pride in work for the staff. These aspirations are not left for us to guess what they might mean operationally. The trust spells this out (Box 3.1).

Box 3.1 Making value tokenism a myth

Best possible care:

- Services that are *safe*, in which there are no needless deaths.
- Services that are *effective*, in which there is no needless pain.
- Services that are *timely*, in which there are no delays.
- Services that are *efficient*, in which there is no waste.
- Services that are *equitable*, in which there are no inequalities.
- Services that are *patient-centred*, in which there are no feelings of helplessness.

Improved health:

- We will treat the whole person, respecting emotional, psychological and spiritual needs, not just the physical.
- We will act in partnership with other providers of health and social care, with patients, their families, their representatives and with the wider local community.
- We will work to reduce inequalities in health status.
- We will play our part in improving health and the outcomes of care for the local population and the people who use our services.

Joy and pride in work:

- We will set clear objectives and expectations for staff.
- We will invest in their training and development.
- We will ensure that staff receive feedback and appreciation for their efforts.
- We will value good, open and honest communication at all levels.
- We will ensure that staff are fairly rewarded.
- We will empower staff to effect change.

The trust makes value tokenism a myth by clearly setting out how it delivers its aspirations. It does this through seven supporting strategies:

- To make patients and their carers full partners in developing and delivering services, involving them in all that we do.
- To place the improvement of quality and safety at the heart of our services.
- To recruit, retain, develop and motivate highly skilled and committed staff.
- To have first-class management and leadership throughout the organisation.
- To use the benefits of IT to deliver better services.
- To have a capital infrastructure that is fit for purpose.
- To establish effective partnerships with local health and social care providers and commissioners of our service.

Value conquest

This is where one value, or set of values, effectively makes some staff reluctantly surrender their value(s). This process is related closely to issues of power, influence and persuasion. It also has a great deal to do with the influence of central government policy and how far staff perceive this to be imposed upon them.

Value alienation

This is another kind of problem for healthcare professionals. It is where values begin to be articulated, by some, which run counter to strongly held personal values. Alienation also arises when personal and collective standards are compromised by influences that staff feel are beyond their control. Common examples of this kind of alienation are related to giving patients quality time when what we feel is valued is 'getting the paperwork right', between maintaining the highest possible standards of care in a context of financial stringency and pervasive values of greater efficiency and even more for less, and between the pressures for effective and fast patient through-flow against patient need and safety.

Value conflict

This can be a nasty organisational virus, eroding and undermining all those things that make a team and make the organisation the kind of place it is. Value conflicts may be concerned with clashes, impasse, getting stuck and staying stuck. For example, one team member may passionately believe that patients should be involved fully and consulted in all aspects of their care, because everyone has the fundamental right to self-determination; other members may take issue with this, and the conflict may show in their actions. For example, operations may be explained hastily to patients, parents and family, with diagrams drawn on scraps of paper. The impression given is that informing patients and significant others, and gaining their consent to treatment, is something of a chore. Another example of value conflict might be concerned with those members who actively wish to promote patient choice, with dignity and justice in mind, and those who hold other views. Value conquest, alienation and conflict at the individual and collective level are a real source of disaffection, low morale and stress. Together, they are a major reason why staff members leave their jobs. They erode any sense that 'this is a great place to work'.

Espoused values and values-in-action

For this to be a successful pathway-to-scale, there has to be a genuine understanding, within organisations, of the need for congruence between what is said (espoused values) and what is done (values-in-action). Put another way, it is not enough for r-learning to be 'talked up' and regarded as a good thing. R-learning has to be seen to be done. It has to be valued in this way, to be done systematically, rigorously and publicly. This is the only way benefits will become known and be observable. We need to strive to achieve an overt behavioural alignment between espoused values and values-in-action. Although this may not always be achievable, it is a goal. The business of knowing, espousing and trying to put values into action has been helpfully and provocatively explored by the many writings of Jack Whitehead from the University of Bath, UK (Whitehead 1993, 2000, Whitehead, with Johns 2000). Readers may also find it helpful to consult Whitehead's website and explore his thoughtful and relevant ideas about viewing ourselves as a living contradiction when our values are negated in our practice and the notion of 'living theory' (www.bath.ac. uk/~edsajw). These are challenging ideas and putting anything into practice, living through our values, might feel impossible some days in healthcare. We need courage to reflect on the alignment between what we say and do. R-learning might usefully be seen as a catalyst that (re-)creates positive (inter)actions between our values, with the best interests of service users in mind.

Linking convictions with actions

Our espoused values are what we say. They are our articulated convictions. They are what we are passionate about, for example convictions about what constitutes 'good practice', about what works in the best interests of patients, and about what makes a particular clinical area a compelling place in which to work. Espoused values are what we promote. For example, the mantra of the incoming UK Labour government in 1997 was 'Education! Education! Education!' From 2001 it has been 'Delivery! Delivery! Delivery!' This has been associated with a raft of NHS reforming and modernising values (and actions). So, values can be positive things. The trick is to know how best to link these convictions with our actions, and in so doing amplify the positive. Sometimes what we say, or espouse, is different from what we do. Sometimes this is inevitable, given the circumstances. If 'greatness is not a function of circumstance' but 'largely a matter of conscious choice and discipline' (Collins 2006, p. 31), then the values we choose and the disciplined ways we try to put them into action (how we operationalise them) are worth reflecting upon. In much public-sector work, 'performance relative to mission is the primary definition of success' (Collins 2006, p. 32). Put another way, performance (action) relative to the values we espouse (mission) is the primary definition of success. This is a challenge. Davies (2002) offers us an insight into the nature of such a challenge. In a paper titled 'Understanding organizational culture in reforming the National Health Service', he writes:

> ... what emerges from evaluations of large-scale structural reforms is how little they impact below surface manifestations. Organisational structures are changed, new names and job titles emerge, the rhetoric and jargon adapt to

new expectations, but service realities often remain stubbornly resistant to change. The central paradox then is why, with more cash and radical reorganisation, does so little change? Those interested in 'complex systems' have no difficulty in understanding the lack of responsiveness: they see such 'non-linearity' (large stimulus, small response) as integral to systems as complex as the NHS (Plsek & Wilson 2001). However, another way of unravelling the paradox is to ask a different question: what are the structures that matter the most – those formal and explicit structures of organisational charts, accountability relationships and contracts? Or the psychological and social structuring that govern how we think, what we value and what we see as legitimate? Much of health system reform has tackled the former, while much that impedes change is concerned with the latter. These informal structures within an organisation – are sometimes referred to as 'the software of the mind' (Hofstede 1994).

(Davies 2002, p. 140)

Espoused theory and theory-in-use

What I have just written does not simply signify the difference between what people say and do. For example, Argyris & Schön (1978) suggest that there is a theory consistent with what people say and a theory consistent with what they do. Therefore, the distinction is not between theory and action, but between two different 'theories of action' (Argyris *et al.* 1985, p. 82), hence the terms 'espoused theory' and 'theory-in-use'. The former consists of the values upon which people believe their behaviour is based. The latter are the values implied by their behaviour, or the convictions they use to take and justify their action. They suggest that people are often unaware that their theories-in-use are not the same as their espoused theories. This raises the question: If people are unaware of the theories that drive their action (their theories-in-use), how can they effectively manage their behaviour? And if they cannot manage their own behaviour, then how can they claim to effectively manage the behaviours of others? This is not only a question for NHS managers and leaders, but for everyone. If behaviours are predicated upon how we feel and think, another question arises: If we cannot manage these, how can we claim to be effective healthcare practitioners? There is a suggestion embedded in this point, namely that an awareness of the power and relevance of emotional intelligence, in healthcare work, is a must for all.

Argyris & Schön (1974) developed a model in order to show how our theories-in-use are created, maintained and changed. It contains the following parts:

- *Governing variables:* These are our values. We usually have more than one of them. The action we take impacts upon a number of these variables simultaneously.
- *Action strategies:* These are the strategies we use to keep our governing values within an acceptable range – in other words, strategies that

enable us to put our values into action and not compromise or distort them in so doing.

- *Consequences:* The strategies we use have two kinds of consequence, intended and unintended.

An example may help to illustrate this process. A recently appointed modern matron talked to me about her core value of respecting the wishes of all her staff. This was one of her governing variables. In any given situation, it is likely that she would design action strategies to keep this governing variable (value) within acceptable limits. These limits were defined by her personal standards of human interaction, her professional codes of conduct, human resources trust policies about dignity at work, bullying, and so on. On one occasion, and in the company of some nursing staff, a conflict arose over the off-duty rota. She avoided addressing the conflict and said as little as possible. In a reflective conversation later, she disclosed to me that this avoidance (she hoped) would suppress the conflict. She claimed that this strategy would allow her to appear to be acting in line with her espoused value. 'Well, at least I didn't say anything wrong, did I?' This strategy had various consequences, both for her and for the nurses involved. Her intended consequence was that the nurses involved would eventually 'give up bickering and arguing'. The intention was that her strategy of non-intervention would successfully diffuse the conflict. But by saying little, by listening and by not intervening, she left herself open to being seen as incompetent and weak by some of her nursing staff. The unintended consequence (brought more into perspective through her reflective conversation) was that she felt the situation had been left unresolved and therefore likely to recur. She felt dissatisfied.

Developing our competence

We can see that there are a number of elements to Argyris & Schön's (1974) model that help to explain how we link our thoughts and actions. These elements are:

- governing variables (or values);
- action strategies;
- intended and unintended consequences for ourselves;
- intended and unintended consequences for others involved;
- action strategy effectiveness.

This simple model has big implications for the way we develop our competence. The consequences of any action may be intended or unintended. When the consequences of the action strategy employed are as we intend, then there is a match (or constructive alignment) between intention and outcome. When this situation occurs, our theory-in-use is confirmed. But if the consequences are unintended and run counter to satisfying our governing values, there is a mismatch between intention and outcome. Argyris and Schön (1974) suggest that we may respond to such a mismatch in one of two ways: through a process of single-loop or double-loop learning. Argyris *et al.* (1985) suggest that the first response to a mismatch between intention and outcome is to search for another action strategy that will satisfy the governing variable(s). For example, the modern matron might intervene sensitively next time, being careful to assess the merits of the different points of view being expressed, and doing so in a balanced way. Here, the new action strategy is used in order to satisfy the existing governing variable (respecting the wishes of all her staff). The change is in the action only, not in the governing variable itself. Such a process is called single-loop learning.

Another possible response would be for the modern matron to reflect upon, modify or change her governing value (respecting the wishes of all her staff). Through her associated action strategies of engaging in a reflective conversation, and being more open with her colleagues, she decided to modify this value and make explicit, for herself, why she was doing this. She modified it to 'openly showing respect for all her staff through what she said and did'. This was her modified conviction. She felt this was more appropriate, achievable and professional. Therefore, in this case, both the governing variable *and* the action strategy changed. This constitutes what is called double-loop learning.

The moral courage to put values-into-action

It takes courage to try to put our values into action. We need to understand the root causes when we are successful in doing this and reflect upon where, and why, there may be contradictions between what we say and do. So why is courage important? It cannot be important for its own sake, because terrorists and murderers, for example, may have courage. In order to think of courage as a virtue, we need an adjective to go alongside it. For example, we could think about moral courage, because there is also amoral courage. Kidder (2005) puts it like this: Moral courage is a phrase that refers

> . . . to a courage that operates within the realm of concern for good and bad, right and wrong. But if by moral we mean that which is good, then moral courage also means the positive courage to be ethical . . . And if by ethical we mean taking action that accords with the core values of honesty, fairness, respect, responsibility and compassion, then moral courage means the courage to invoke the practice of those values . . . And if the word values is in some way synonymous with convictions, then moral courage is, as it's often characterised, 'the courage of our convictions' in these five key areas.

(Kidder 2005, pp. 69–70)

Without courage, our values become inoperative. Even the most sophisticated and beautifully written values need to be made active. What use is a conviction such as 'we treat everyone with respect and dignity' without an ability and willingness to put this value into action?

Without the courage to act, virtuous convictions in the form of trust-wide values are pointless.

Values-into-action: things get in the way

Sometimes this is easier said than done. Sometimes things get in the way of a simple application of values into action. These 'intervening variables' may be operational, strategic, cultural, philosophical, ideological or pragmatic. They may have something to do with time, resources (financial and human), communication, history, expectations, energy, and so on. One approach that might affect the process of values-into-action is that which focuses on the practical consequences of what we might do. Another concentrates on the actions themselves. This reflects the two traditions in modern philosophical ethics regarding how to determine the ethical character of actions. One argues that actions have no intrinsic ethical character but acquire their moral status from the consequences that flow from them. The other tradition claims that actions are inherently right or wrong, such as lying, cheating and stealing. The former is called a teleological approach, the latter deontological.

Ends-oriented

The first approach (ends-oriented) is particularly appealing to some because it takes a pragmatic and common-sense approach to action. Put simply, teleological thinkers claim that the moral character of actions depends on the simple, practical matter of the extent to which actions actually help or hurt people. Actions that produce more benefits than harm are 'right'; those that do not are 'wrong.' This approach is often regarded as utilitarian and is a school of thought originated by the British thinker Jeremy Bentham (1748–1832) and refined by John Stuart Mill (1806–73). In the context of healthcare, it is an approach that encourages us to focus on trying to arrive at good (clinical) outcomes and results. The central weakness of the Bentham–Mill approach to action is that as long as an action or policy produces enough 'good outcomes', any action is theoretically defensible. As we can imagine, in healthcare this is a matter of considerable debate. Put another way, the outcome justifies the means. But what outcome, and for whom? The common-sense appeal of this approach is seductive. A careful analysis of means and ends is needed. Also, the immediate and longer-term consequences of the outcomes for all involved, and the astute discernment of the nature and quality of any alternative means and outcomes, if indeed there are any, need to be reflected on. The greatest good for the greatest number doesn't promise good for everyone. The approach simply urges us to maximise the good, even if some may be harmed.

Act-oriented

The second approach (act-oriented) is based on an idea that teleological thinkers flatly deny, namely that actions have intrinsic moral value. Some actions are considered inherently good (truth-telling, keeping promises, respecting the rights of patients), while others are bad (dishonesty, coercion, manipulation, exploitation). No matter how much good might come from being disrespectful, argues a deontological thinker, the action will never be right. So the only question of importance is: Which actions are inherently good? Instead of engaging in complex projections about the consequences of some action, this approach focuses simply on the nature of the action itself. For example, in healthcare, it means: Does it respect the basic human rights of everyone involved? Does the action avoid deception, coercion and manipulation? Does it treat people equally and fairly, with dignity and respect? The most representative deontological thinker is Immanuel Kant (1724–1804). Kant believed that he discovered the fundamental law that would determine the ethical character of any action, without regard to its consequences. Kant called this law the 'categorical imperative', in other words something that holds no matter what the circumstances. It was derived from reason itself and from a belief that we are free, rational and moral agents. Kant claimed that the only thing inherently good was a 'good will' and that this comes from a sense of duty. A good will chooses what it does simply and purely because it is the right thing to do, not because it is inclined to do some deed, nor because it has positive consequences. In healthcare, this approach encourages us to reflect upon the basic idea that consequences are irrelevant, that we cannot judge the value of any action by (only) assessing how it turned out. From whistle-blowing, which some advocate, to the most principled and selfless of clinical actions, these and others can produce fatal and hugely damaging outcomes. Perhaps the main difficulty with using this approach in healthcare is its inflexibility. If lying (or being economical with the truth) is intrinsically wrong, then there is no way to justify it even when it produces more good than harm. This lack of compromise makes this approach a challenging one to live by.

The principle of reciprocity

There is a third approach, which may be helpful in healthcare. This approach arguably lies somewhere between the teleological and deontological approaches. It is one that encourages us to think about our actions from the perspective of what we would want others to do to us. It is based upon the *principle of reciprocity* and invites us to imagine that we are in another's shoes, about to be affected by the very actions we are contemplating. If we cannot say confidently that the action we are about to take towards another would be acceptable if taken towards us (me), then this may be a moment to stop and reflect upon the ethical character of what we are about to do. Again, there is much to reflect upon here and encapsulated in the phrase 'Do to others as you would have them do to you'. Who are these 'others'? Clearly, the application of these approaches does not automatically produce 'the answer'. Codes of conduct and duties of care intersect with them. Maybe they tug us in different directions, in different circumstances. Maybe for you they blur along their edges. In your health-care work, which of your values have intrinsic worth and would you wish others to hold and follow, regardless of the consequences? For other values you may have, what are the consequences of putting them into action? Is the whole issue of values-into-action more a matter of conscience or consequence for you? What are the risks of one or the other?

Building a reflective organisation means that a critical mass of staff needs to subscribe to the following value: to engage in collaborative forms of r-learning and doing this in a systematic, supported, rigorous and public manner. Progress along this action pathway symbolises progress towards building a reflective organisation.

Action pathway: conversation

During 2006, the Institute of Reflective Practice-UK was asked to run a series of one-day team-building events for groups of up to 25 staff in maternity services for a large UK strategic health authority. These events formed part of an ongoing service improvement project. They were attended by midwives, healthcare support workers, administrative and support staff, nurses, scientists, technicians, therapists, managers and, occasionally, a consultant. The starting point for each trust was 'team-building'. The starting point for the Institute was to try to build a conversation around service improvement that was creative, hopeful and optimistic. Institute staff made this clear to each trust. These two positions were not seen as incompatible. On one of the days, a short but hugely significant exchange of views, started by two senior midwives, went like this:

> **Simone:** *It's not that we don't meet to discuss and reflect on our work. We do. In fact, we talk a lot. Don't we? In every meeting, we talk, talk, talk. We seem to talk quite openly.*
> **Una:** Yes, but most of our talk doesn't seem to change anything.

> **Simone:** *I agree with you. But why do we feel like this?*
> **Una:** Well, I think it's because we talk mostly about our problems. It's just problem talk. My feeling is that the more we talk about them, the more depressed we become. Well, I do anyway. If anyone listened to our meetings, they'd think that all we do is talk to each other about problems.

> **Simone:** *But these are real and important. We have to. We can't just ignore them, can we?*
> **Una:** No. But the more we do this [talk about problems], the more fed up we get. Sometimes I've left our meetings thinking that we've got a bigger problem at the end than we had at the beginning. We just seem to go on unravelling it. You know, like the onion skin.

> **Simone:** *Are you saying we shouldn't talk about problems then?*
> **Una:** No. What I'm trying to say is, what's a better way of talking to each other?

> **Simone:** *A better way?*
> **Una:** Yes. A different way . . . that's better. A more positive one.

The problem of focusing on problems

This sparked off a lengthy discussion. Two things (initially) emerged from this. The first was an insight; the second was a question. The insight was that the more they felt they were focusing on 'their problems', the more the problems seemed to grow in magnitude, significance to them and detail. The longer this went on, the more drained and frustrated they became. They appreciated that their problem talk was often linked with 'solutions'. For example, if 'the problem' was a shortage of staff, then the discussion narrowed down and focused on ways of increasing staff numbers (the solution). The question that emerged was: 'What would it take for us to feel we can really move forward?' Coupled with this was an appreciation that their existing team meetings were organised entirely around talking and that this talk was dominated by those who were sufficiently confident and articulate to speak up. They were characterised as 'noisy meetings'. I discovered that a lack of turn-taking skills meant that more than one person spoke at once, so some could talk but there were issues around listening, in other words actively being able to take something in, mull it over and respond appropriately. The enormous potential within this group of staff to discuss new and different ways forward was being underutilised. For many people, it is not problems that energise them, but discussions about possibilities for (even) better care, discussions about what is valued and desired, 'What if?' conversations. As problems grow in size, so our optimism wanes. So what stops us having more discussions that explore positive experiences that focus on discovering, in the past, the root causes of our success and then asking ourselves the questions 'How can we (re-)create conditions where we can repeat this (or appropriate features of this) success now?' and 'If we have experienced this once, so we know it's achievable, what's stopping us doing it again?'

Part way through this discussion, another midwife, in a quiet and considered manner said:

> I don't think we can solve our problems unless people talk more openly, honestly and respectfully to each other. We can't have messages left for us on the ward, where our manager talks to us as if we were children. We can't have her [another senior manager] giving us a PowerPoint presentation on being respectful to each other, when she's the biggest bully of them all. We can only have these different kinds of meetings when we learn to listen without judging . . . listen to what we all have to say . . . to offer . . . Then we might hear something new. We might discover something we haven't thought about . . . what's possible. If we want to give better care to our women, and I think we all do, then we might have to learn to change ourselves, act differently towards each other. I mean, when was the last time you got a thankyou from another member of staff? Today . . . no. Yesterday . . . again, no. So when, and why not? I can't understand it, and it's depressing. I feel we always see each other as roles, not as people, don't you? I mean, we don't even know everyone's first name today, and it's not that any of us have just started working here. I think to do a really

good job for our clients, we need each other. So why can't we change things? Things won't change for us by themselves. We'll have to do something. But what can we do? I'll shut up now . . . I've said too much anyway. Sorry.

If we don't act, nothing will ever change

These thoughts and feelings were greeted with spontaneous applause from many in the room. It was like the lid had been taken off something. The midwife smiled and a tear ran down her face. Others comforted her. In this one moment, everything changed. The atmosphere in the room changed. The expressions on people's faces changed. Staff began to relate to each other in a reassuring and giving manner. They wanted to begin talking to one another again, differently and more meaningfully. More staff wanted to tell their own stories. More were willing to listen. They wanted to share their own concerns and struggles. Many said they felt alone even though they were working in a busy unit. It took just one person to have the courage to begin a different kind of conversation. And what emerged was that others were just waiting for someone else to start it. Perhaps they weren't quite as brave as the midwife who did speak. But perhaps the greatest source of courage is to appreciate that if we do not act, then nothing will ever change for the better. This midwife's action created a 'tipping point'. It 'tipped' the rest of the day away from valuing problems to valuing each other, away from problems and towards successes, away from what staff felt they wanted to get rid of (problems) and towards what they felt they wanted more of (more trust, respect and feelings of positive regard). Although there was a tendency across the rest of the day to slide back into problem talk, what emerged was a feeling that keeping the balance of the conversation 'tipped' towards strengths and successes required some new work habits and mental discipline. Much of this was around having the confidence to let go of service problems (deficit-based conversations) and (re-)learn a vocabulary that would sustain new strength-based conversations.

An understanding of the idea of the tipping point

In his international bestseller *The Tipping Point*, Gladwell (2005) reminds us of the way little things can make a big difference. This is encapsulated within his book. He also suggests that the best way to understand how ideas and innovations spread, how work habits emerge, ebb and flow, is to see them as epidemics. 'Ideas and products and messages and behaviours spread just like viruses do' (Gladwell 2005, p. 7). His main thesis is like this: First, we need to expose a few people to a new idea or way of doing things, for example encouraging staff to think more about and understand better the roots of success and than the root causes of failures. This 'infects' them with the success 'virus'. These people then start acting differently. Second, this small change (for example, through a one-day workshop) has a big impact on others. Somehow the effect is dramatic. Staff go away and talk to others about the day, how it has made them feel, how challenging but how uplifting they found it. Third, this does not happen slowly but in a hurry – maybe in one moment, in one action. It may be because of a chance meeting, a reaction to an email, a timely conversation during team briefing, at a handover, during a conference presentation, in the coffee room or sluice. Anywhere, any time, things can 'tip'.

Gladwell illustrates each of the following three characteristics:

- contagiousness;
- a little input, of a certain kind, can have a big effect;
- change can happen dramatically and in one moment.

He argues that it is the third characteristic that is the most important to understand as it helps us to make sense of the first two. The one dramatic moment when everything can change, all at once (as in the example above), is what he calls the 'Tipping Point'. In a cash-strapped health service, or one where there never seems to be sufficient time to do what we want and need to do properly, understanding how we get things to 'tip' seems very useful. So what would some of the highly (and positively) contagious ideas be in your organisation? R-learning, if described, explained and justified in the ways suggested in Figure 0.2 on p. 15 might, for some, have this property. Contagiousness is about something 'catching on'. For this to happen, staff have to be exposed to r-learning in some appropriate manner. The second characteristic means that we have to move away from thinking about proportionality. What we put into r-learning must be related directly, in spread and impact, to what comes out. Gladwell (2005) argues that we need to prepare ourselves for the possibility that sometimes big changes follow from small events. This is a change in mindset.

The possibility of sudden change is at the heart of the idea of the tipping point. In healthcare, we might wish to ask:

- Why is it that some ideas and processes start epidemics (in Gladwell's sense) and others don't?
- What can we do to deliberately start and sustain positive social epidemics such as r-learning?
- Is there more than one way to tip something?

Gladwell states:

Epidemics are a function of the people who transmit infectious agents, the infectious agent itself, and the environment in which the infectious agent is operating. And when an epidemic tips, when it is jolted out of equilibrium, it tips because something has happened.

(Gladwell 2005, pp. 18–19)

In other words, some change has occurred in one or more of the characteristics described above. Gladwell goes on to suggest that using the idea of the tipping point, in our own organisations, requires us to understand three change agents:

- the Law of the Few;
- the Stickiness Factor;
- the Power of Context.

Applying these ideas to building a reflective healthcare organisation could have these implications. The Law of the Few means that r-learning is likely to be driven by the efforts of a handful of exceptional people – exceptional in the sense of how energetic they are, how knowledgeable of r-learning they are, how enthusiastic they are about it and how influential they are among their peers. Concentrating this building process on a few key people seems prudent. This is a conscious, high-impact strategy. It is also a positive step towards getting the process of r-learning to tip. In addition, we have to get two more things right:

- *Word-of-mouth processes:* This means what staff actually say about r-learning is important. A key question then becomes: Which values and processes might tip r-learning so that it becomes a sustainable, organisation-wide, positive work habit, and which won't?
- *The involvement of people:* The choice of who are the 'few', the advocate(s), and what constitutes the 'few', appears to be a critical one.

An understanding of the importance of stickiness in tipping has enormous implications for the way we might build a reflective healthcare organisation. Gladwell puts it this way:

> We tend to spend a lot of time thinking about how to make messages more contagious – how to reach as many people as possible with our products or ideas. But the hard part of communication is often figuring out how to make sure a message doesn't go in one ear and out the other. Stickiness means that a message makes an impact. You can't get it out of your head. It sticks in your memory.

(Gladwell 2005, pp. 24–5)

So what might be the 'stickiness' of r-learning? What can we do or say to make r-learning more memorable? How we manage the word-of-mouth process is a part of this. The 'few' need to be information brokers. This includes the ability of those involved to share and trade knowledge about the nature and benefits of r-learning. In discharging this role, it helps if they know a wide range of staff. So the 'few' also need to be connectors; by this, I mean they need to be able to bring staff together and be able to persuade sceptical colleagues, through word and deed, of the benefits of r-learning. By implication, then, they need to be salespeople. A key question then becomes 'What makes someone persuasive, and can we find such people inside our organisations?'

It may not be possible to find all these qualities in one person. Whatever the case, my point is that building a reflective organisation requires brokers (who provide the right messages), connectors (who provide the social glue) and salespeople (who get staff to actively buy-in to the benefits of r-learning). If we spend too much time on spreading the word about r-learning and reaching as many staff as possible, there is a danger that insufficient time will be spent on making the values and processes of r-learning stick. Put simply, in the busyness of working life, if staff fail to remember what it is we want them to know about r-learning, then their heads, hands and hearts won't change. The message has to be memorable.

Getting healthcare conversations to tip

In Fig. 3.2 I characterise six different kinds of conversation that we have inside healthcare organisations. There are more of course, and some are more familiar than others. I suggest that the two conversations on the left are essentially conversations about what we may want less of. The two on the right are what we may want more of. The two in the middle represent different kinds of reflective learning – one I call 'critical', the other 'appreciative'. Both relate to arguments I have advanced (see action step 1). In Fig. 3.2 I have attempted to link the kinds of conversation we might have with particular kinds of organisational mindscapes. I suggest that a purpose of Fig. 3.2 is in its role as a catalyst for a conversation, among staff, about dominant organisational discourses and how changing the way we talk might help us change the way we work.

Figure 3.3 is suggesting that at any one time, our conversations may tip to the right or to the left (no party political message is being given here). When conversations tip left, those involved recognise that an amplification of the problem is necessary. A tip to the right means that an amplification of a particular success is appropriate. A reflective organisation generates both deficit- and strength-based conversations according to the exigencies of the moment. They are, in other words, 'situated' conversations. Staff working in a reflective organisation are fully aware when they have (and need) to amplify 'problems' or their 'successes'.

Using the power of the positive question

How can we shift the balance of healthcare conversations that are stuck with vocabularies of human deficit and, in so doing, unlock the creative potential of staff inside organisations? I ask this because we know that deficit-based questions lead to deficit-based conversations, which in turn lead to deficit-based patterns of action (Anderson *et al.* 2006, Cooperrider and Whitney 2005). So how do we address this constructively? I suggest that if we ask different kinds of question, then we are likely to generate different kinds of conversation.

Advocates of appreciative enquiry (Cooperrider & Whitney 1999, Cooperrider *et al.* 2003, 2005, Srivastva *et al.* 1990, Whitney & Trosten-Bloom 2002, Whitney *et al.* 2002, 2005) talk a lot about the *power of the*

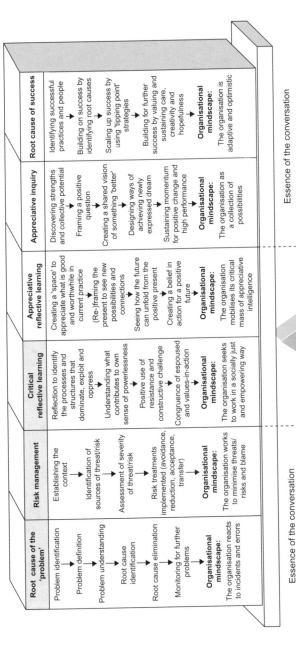

Figure 3.2 Spectrum of conversations within a reflective organisation.

Root cause of the 'problem'	Risk management	Critical reflective learning	Appreciative reflective learning	Appreciative inquiry	Root cause of success
Problem identification	Establishing the context	Reflection to identify the processes and structures that dominate, exploit and oppress	Creating a 'space' to appreciate what is good and worthwhile in current practice	Discovering strengths and collective potential	Identifying successful practices and people
Problem definition	Identification of sources of threat/risk	Understanding what contributes to own sense of powerlessness	(Re-)framing the present to see new possibilities and connections	Framing a positive question	Building on success by identifying root causes
Problem understanding	Assessment of severity of threat/risk	Positive use of resistance and constructive challenge	Seeing how the future can unfold from the positive present	Creating a shared vision of something 'better'	Scaling up success by using 'tipping point' strategies
Root cause identification	Risk treatments implemented (avoidance, reduction, acceptance, transfer)	Congruence of espoused and values-in-action	Creating a belief in action for a positive future	Designing ways of achieving newly expressed dream	Building for further success by valuing and sustaining care, creativity and hopefulness
Root cause elimination				Sustaining momentum for positive change and high performance	
Monitoring for further problems					
Organisational mindscape: The organisation reacts to incidents and errors	**Organisational mindscape:** The organisation works to minimise threats/ risks and blame	**Organisational mindscape:** The organisation seeks to work in a socially just and empowering way	**Organisational mindscape:** The organisation mobilises its critical mass of appreciative intelligence	**Organisational mindscape:** The organisation as a collection of possibilities	**Organisational mindscape:** The organisation is adaptive and optimistic

Tipping point

Essence of the conversation

Drilling down, searching for certainty and the truth on the matter

'What we want less of is ...' (minimising strategies)

Appreciating when to let go of the 'problem' and how to welcome in new possibilities for action

Essence of the conversation

Opening up in pursuit of possibilities for working positively with uncertainty and ambiguity in order to improve services and workplaces

'What we want more of is ...' (maximising strategies)

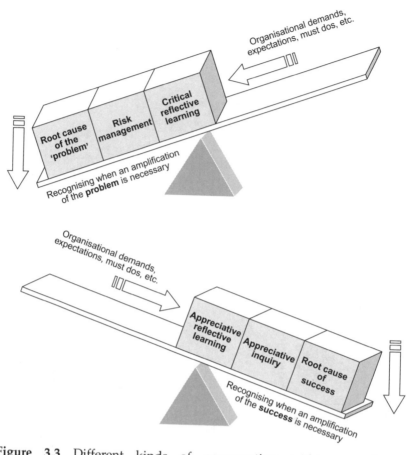

Figure 3.3 Different kinds of conversation within a reflective organisation.

positive question. This question guides agendas and focuses organisational attention in the direction of the aspects of organisational existence – latent or explicit, historic or contemporary – that are most life-giving and life-sustaining for employees. It is a kind of question that enables the creation of powerful vocabularies of possibility, both in the day-to-day conversations of staff and in the social and organisational theory that is produced about service improvement and workplace transformation.

Because of the centrality of the positive question to the building of a reflective healthcare organisation, I first want to raise a few contextual issues before giving a practical example of a question of this kind. Gergen (1994) argues that we should be very wary of what he calls 'critical scholarship' and more generally 'critique' of all kinds. This is particularly relevant to my earlier points about deficit-based conversations and more generally critical forms of reflective practice (see action step 1).

Gergen raises five consequences of conversations of this kind. I have interpreted them thus:

- *Containment of conversation:* Deficit-based conversations, as I have presented them, often operate to establish a dualistic conversational structure in which this is opposed to that. For example, let's assume the argument is that flatter forms of organisational structure and sending home, after 24 hours, a low-risk woman who has had a normal delivery and healthy baby are good things. Deficit-based conversations tend to lock us into a 'flatter form/not a flatter form' or 'send home/don't send home' linguistic structure. This is, by its very nature, conservative because it confines conversation within this dualism. Words, sentences, images and ideas that lie outside of the dualism tend to be ignored.
- *Silencing of other voices:* Once this kind of conversational dualism is established, it brings with it another problem: it tends to silence other, alternative points of view. For example, conversations about male medical dominance simultaneously serve to reify a distinction between men and women. When conversations about different healthcare disciplines are couched in the language of turf, territory and conflict, a conversation around difference is sustained. Because the conversation tends to proceed within the terms of the dualism, other realities, values and concerns are removed from earshot.
- *Search for deficiencies:* Once locked into the two points above, deficit-based conversations are usually sustained by an array of 'what we want less of' and 'catch you out'-type questions, a search for certainty and 'truth', and questions that try to expose others and debunk the accounts of those speaking in another way. As a result, conversations with 'others' (other colleagues/staff) tend to slide into an intentional and rigorous search for others' most glaring deficits, deficiencies and weaknesses. Human wholeness and complexity get lost. The notion of multiple and constructed realities also gets lost.
- *Fragmentation of relationships:* It's no surprise that the posture of those who may, for example, be attending a team meeting and who constantly live through deficit-based conversations, is anything other than defensive and disappointed. The energy that is put into reacting to incidents and errors, trying to minimise risk, and apportioning responsibility and blame serves only to fragment teams and destroy cohesion. It demoralises and separates. It drives wedges between people rather than bonding them together.
- *Negative workplace cultures:* Everything I have said has an impact on workplace cultures. When we have staff who tend to talk more about problems than possibilities, failures instead of successes, then a culture of negativity can be created. Staff tend to close ranks around preferred ways of talking and interacting. This re-affirms their relationships, their value positions and their solidarity.

Aspects of lived experience

A positive question is one that invites staff to reflect upon and then to give voice to those aspects of their lived experience (van Manen 1997) that gives them a sense of joy, fulfilment and satisfaction in their work and workplace. By asking positive questions, we give ourselves a chance to create powerful vocabularies of possibility, in particular thinking about the possibility of positively re-experiencing past successes and doing more of what satisfies and achieves agreed goals. In a reflective organisation, asking positive questions is a daily work habit. This habit embraces two fundamental conceptions of reflection, namely the acts of looking back and looking forward – looking back and rediscovering joys, excellence and innovation, and then looking forward and asking the positive question 'What single thing, were it to happen again and *more frequently*, would make a significant and positive difference to my work here?' When I invite groups to reflect upon this question, there is usually much discussion around the inclusion of 'more frequently' and how omitting it changes everything about the sentence. The phrase 'significant and positive' is also a cause of much debate. I invited a multidisciplinary team working in a maternity unit to write down their responses to this question. Box 3.2 shows some of their responses.

Box 3.2   Some responses to the positive question 'What single thing, were it to happen again and *more frequently*, would make a significant and positive difference to my work here?'

- I'd like my skills to be recognised again and would want to get back those feelings of being supported, so that I can function to my maximum capacity.
- What was wonderful was the way we shared our workload with colleagues, if they were busier than you were. I want this sharing to happen more frequently.
- I loved it when everyone had a positive attitude of work commitment and worked to the same goal.
- I remember when I was treated like a human being. As a human being I was appreciated and respected. What I want more frequently is to feel appreciated, which will help me perform to my best ability.
- Happen again and more frequently . . . to be treated with respect.
- I've worked here for 18 years and I can recall when people were recognised for what they did. It was a time when people had respect for one another, speaking or supporting one another when things went wrong. Somehow we need to have more of this.
- More acknowledgement and thanks for your hard work and continued commitment. It happens, but we could do with more of this. It's all about feeling good.

(Continued)

- I have experienced what it's like to be part of a team that had the ability to listen and I had the 'right' to be listened to. We need more democratic listening to happen more frequently.
- More *appreciation* for one another, more frequently. I used to work in a positive environment. What made it like that was that we appreciated each other. So can we get more of this going again?
- We are not really any bigger now, and back then we communicated effectively. We did this because we spoke directly to each other. We did it then, so surely we can communicate effectively with everybody now, can't we?
- We met regularly and it worked wonders for teamworking and morale. Also, we all knew what was going on. I would like, within this department, to have more frequent staff meetings, where individual colleagues can be encouraged to project positive changes to improve morale and team building.
- It's simple. I do feel appreciated, by some. But we need to be appreciated more frequently by our managers (management).
- If everybody that I met, each day, smiled and acknowledged me and I them, it would make a significant difference to work here.
- Be greeted by smiling faces who say 'Hello' and 'How are you?' We used to do this more and the place seemed much happier.
- More days like today, encouraging staff to flourish. We had more staff development days then, and we always seemed to feel more positive about our work and able to cope with new demands.

What are we learning?

How can positive questions dislodge the certainty of existing deficit constructions of reality, create spaces for new voices and languages to emerge, build more supportive relational contexts for staff and build a positive construction of social reality (Cooperrider 2001, p. 27). Here are some of the ways that Cooperrider suggests using positive questions makes this possible:

- *They release new positive vocabularies:* Positive questions re-focus an organisation's attention away from problems and towards possibilities. By asking positive questions, we invite staff to use words, phrases, sentences and ideas that typically remain uncelebrated or underused in much of what constitutes normal organisational conversation. This has two consequences: 'First, it begins to loosen the hammerlock that patterns of deficit discourse have on the organisation ... Second, because the restrictive grip of deficit vocabularies is loosened, the positive questions immediately boost energy for action within the organisation. People begin to feel a sense of their own authorship within the organisation. They recognize the strengths and resources that they and others bring to their jobs and this enhances their sense of esteem and efficacy for getting things done. It also generates new ideas for action' (Cooperrider 2001, p. 28).

- *They affirm variety of experience and encourage full voice:* If we adopt a social constructionist view, then it follows that language provides the means through which we communicate the sense we make of our worlds. The language we have available to us, to an extent, determines our possibilities for action. Positive vocabularies give us a chance of acting in the world, positively.
- *They help us value others:* Asking positive questions enables us to appreciate what others value and cherish in their work and so, understandably, what they want more, not less, of.
- *They foster relational connections:* Asking a positive question invites staff to reflect upon their practice and to think of something significant to them. As Table 3.2 (p. 203) shows, what emerges are expressions of our core values and commitments. They are essential things that connect us with others.
- *They help build a sense of community:* 'By inviting participants to inquire deeply into the best and most valued aspects of one another's life and work, it immediately creates a context of empathy, care and mutual affirmation' (Cooperrider 2001, p. 31).
- *They can generate social innovation:* Appreciative approaches to work and working life (Cooperrider & Srivastva 1987), of which the positive question is a central feature, 'are based on the constructionist notion that organisations grow and evolve in the direction of their most positive guiding images of the future. When we inquire into our weaknesses and deficiencies, we gain an expert knowledge of what is "wrong" with our organisations, and we may even become proficient problem-solvers, but we do not strengthen our collective capacity to imagine and to build a better future' (Cooperrider 2001, p. 34).

Building a reflective organisation means that we need to:

- create the opportunity; and
- have the ability to use the power of the positive question to strengthen our collective capacity and capability to both imagine and build (even) better services for patients/clients. Progress along this action pathway symbolises progress towards building a reflective organisation.

Action pathway: user

A headline in the *Nursing Times* on 21 November 2006 contained the following rather disturbing words: 'If service users felt listened to, they'd be happier to compromise'. The focus was on mental health. The main concern of the writer was in the form of a question:

Do you ever wonder if the service people receive is really what they are looking for? . . . So why is it that such a huge gulf exists between those who devise and provide the service and those who use it? To put it bluntly, why are service users not receiving the service they want or need? And why, at the same time, are we patting ourselves on the back for being so great at our jobs, and expecting service users to be grateful and buy us big boxes of chocolates? Could it be that we only pay lip service to each other's point of view? . . . Maybe if service users felt truly listened to they'd be happier to compromise in an imperfect system. And maybe if we didn't feel criticised for trying to do our jobs in this imperfect system, we'd be able to truly listen.

(Gadsby 2006, p. 10)

Clearly there is much to reflect upon and to learn from a view such as this, especially in the context of the UK government's patient-led NHS reforms. The NHS Plan requires each NHS trust in England to obtain feedback from patients about their experiences of care. The NHS Patient Survey Programme covers acute trusts, primary care trusts, mental health, ambulance trusts and others. In addition, other surveys focus on the National Service Frameworks for coronary heart disease, stroke and cancer. There are also plans for surveys to examine long-term conditions such as diabetes. Listening to patients' views is recognised as essential to delivering the commitments given in the NHS Plan to provide a patient-centred health service. The survey results are used in the annual performance indicators published by the Healthcare Commission.

In this section, I suggest that progress along this particular action pathway is essentially about working towards clearly demonstrating the value of being valued. More precisely, becoming a reflective organisation is crucially about scaling up four r-learning processes: building trust with service users, and then engaging with them positively, actively listening to what they have to say, and using the full power of feedback to improve services further. R-learning is needed in order for us to reap the benefit from these processes. I also suggest that we do not simply need more language of valuing. We need to develop the language of positive regard.

The value of being valued

For me, Gadsby's (2006) article is all about the value of being valued, or, more accurately, reflecting systematically and supportively on the benefits of fully valuing service user (and staff) experiences. It seems unwise to me, and especially at a time when the 'system' is under pressure, that we still tend to underuse the communicative channels open to us, to make more widely known the genuinely positive, appreciative and admiring experiences we have of healthcare services. We all do better at work if we regularly have the experience that what we say and do matters, that our presence makes a positive difference to others. With regard to the views of service users, hearing that our work is valued can help confirm, for us, that we matter as a person. It helps us connect with them. Left like this, things are rather lop-sided. We need to actively solicit the views of, and then listen to, service users. I am going to frame such a reciprocal exchange, a conversation of positive regard. But let's be clear: the language of positive regard is not simply about praising, stroking or positively defining a person to him- or herself or to others. In the context of this action pathway, it is to do with having conversations where we become more informed about others' (service users') experiences of the services we manage and deliver. In general, we know that service users' experiences are likely to reflect at least five things:

- their personal preferences;
- their current expectations of the service;
- their personally constructed realities of the care they receive;
- any previous experience(s) of care;
- their current understanding of their future wellbeing.

Attributes of a language of positive regard

So what are some of the key attributes of a language of positive regard? I suggest five to begin. First, it is a language where service users inform us about the *significance* of our services, for them. Second, it is *specific* information about the user's personal experiences. Third, it is *non-attributive*; by this, I mean the conversation focuses on the experience and not on particular members of staff. Fourth, it is potentially *transformational* for both the user and for staff, through the acts of telling and listening. And fifth, such conversations give service users the opportunity to communicate *appreciation*. So we need to ask: What processes are in place in order for a conversation of positive regard to happen? What information is routinely gathered and shared? What is the quality of such conversations? And how far can we be optimistic that such 'patient-centredness' is valued? (see Gerteis *et al.* 1993).

In August 2006, Coulter & Ellins from the Health Foundation and the Picker Institute Europe published a piece of work called *Patient-Focused Interventions: A Review of the Evidence*. Its headline was 'Healthcare policy makers and practitioners disregard patient involvement successes'. The publication collated and analysed evidence published over an eight-year period (1998–2006) into a wide range of patient involvement initiatives worldwide. The report clearly suggests what does and does not work in patient involvement, ranging from patient choice through to self-care and shared decision-making. The lead author and chief executive of the Picker Institute Europe, Professor Angela Coulter, commented in a press release on 16 August 2006:

> Many people want to have a say in decisions about how they are treated, and patient involvement is recognised by the government and professional organisations as an important dimension of patient-centred healthcare. Yet while there is enthusiasm for patient engagement and evidence that it can improve health outcomes, the sector appears slow to adopt and implement these proven strategies.

(Press release, 2006)

Patient-centredness as a critical component of twenty-first-century healthcare

The Picker Institute Europe, which works with patients, professionals and policy-makers to promote understanding of the patient's perspective at all levels of healthcare policy and practice, has identified eight dimensions of patient-centred care from their inpatient surveys. They are:

- *access* (including time spent waiting for admission or time between admission and allocation to a bed in a ward)
- *respect for patients' values, preferences, and expressed needs* (including impact of illness and treatment on quality of life, involvement in decision making, dignity, needs and autonomy)
- *coordination and integration of care* (including clinical care, ancillary and support services, and 'frontline' care)
- *information, communication, and education* (including clinical status, progress and prognosis, processes of care, facilitation of autonomy, self-care and health promotion)
- *physical comfort* (including pain management, help with activities of daily living, surroundings and hospital environment)
- *emotional support and alleviation of fear and anxiety* (including clinical status, treatment and prognosis, impact of illness on self and family, financial impact of illness)
- *involvement of family and friends* (including social and emotional support, involvement in decision making, support for caregiving, impact on family dynamics and functioning)
- *transition and continuity* (including information about medication and danger signals to look out for after leaving hospital, coordination and discharge planning, clinical, social, physical and financial support).

(see www.pickereurope.org/page.php?id=21#pagetop)

Patients as consumers

The notions of a health service that is patient-centred and patient-led reflect certain value positions embedded within UK government reforms. One position is to

> ... enhance the role of patients as 'consumers' of health care, by offering them the right to choose where they receive treatment and by taking other measures designed to make services more responsive to what patients want. However, at the same time, a less overt strand of policy has been emerging. This has focused on a 'citizen' model of patient involvement, in which members of the public (whether or not they are patients at the time) have the right to influence the planning, design and delivery of health care services ... This policy has been pursued through the creation of patient and public involvement forums and, more recently, through developing NHS foundation trusts that are 'owned' by a membership that comprises patients, the wider public and staff.

Foundation trusts have taken public engagement to a new level. They are 'mutual' organisations, where the members have become the legal 'owners' of the hospitals that serve them, or within which they work.

(Lewis *et al.* 2006, p. 6).

Mills (2005) argues that the citizenship approach would appear to provide a basis for NHS reform that keeps the patient at the centre. He goes on to say:

Of equal importance, it might provide a platform to start to address the wider objectives of engaging people in making healthier choices. In the consumerist model, the extent of the user's interest is in securing the service to which they are entitled, whatever the cost. There is no incentive, for example, for those managing long-term conditions to help to reduce the cost of provision, because the result will just be to increase the profitability of the provider. In other words, it is limited by a narrow self-interest. In the citizenship model where the individual is owner and member of the organisation providing the local service, the starting point is a potential relationship with the provider which could encourage the individual to behave differently.

(Mills 2005, p. 13)

Building a language of positive regard through trust

I have argued elsewhere (Ghaye 2005) for the importance of trust for service improvement and workplace transformation initiatives. Although a complex process to establish and sustain, it is usually assumed to be a prerequisite for building shared values, meanings and positive action. Trust is not always easy to achieve, especially where the weight of past betrayals and hostility hangs heavy (Rothstein 2000). However, trust is also made possible precisely by the legacy of the past (Fisman & Khanna 1999, Putnam *et al.* 1993).

Progress along this action pathway towards building a reflective organisation requires us to put some energy and resources into trust building. Without trust, conversations of positive regard are non-starters. Reina & Reina (2006) help us with two things: to appreciate the importance of trust and betrayal in the workplace, and to build trusting relationships. At the heart of their book is the notion of transactional trust. This is a process of mutual exchange, reciprocity and something created incrementally over time. In other words, we have to give trust in order to increase the likelihood that we will receive it. They set out three types of transactional trust:

- *Contractual trust:* This is essentially a trust of character, or, put another way, people actually doing what they say they will do, doing what they promise. It is about keeping agreements, honouring intentions and behaving consistently. In a survey conducted by the Institute of

Reflective Practice-UK as part of an initiative to build and sustain excellence in maternity services in one part of the UK, 1472 women completed a questionnaire and wrote an additional 32 000 words in a free-writing section about their experiences of the services they received. As part of the 'contract', we promised respondents that we would feed back, to as many of them as possible, the major findings of the survey. At the time of writing this book, we have, thus far, done this principally through maternity service liaison committees. We kept our promise to service users. We had to. This appeared to be regarded positively and brought forth comments such as 'This is the first time we have actually got feedback on a survey. Usually we fill in the forms and then we hear nothing more.'

- *Communication trust:* This is essentially a trust of disclosure. Put another way, it is about people's willingness to share information, tell the truth, admit mistakes, celebrate achievements and successes, maintain confidentiality, and give and receive constructive feedback. Trust influences the quality of our conversations, and vice versa. This kind of trust underpins the stated value of a patient-led NHS. If we are to build a reflective organisation, then a secure platform of communication trust is fundamental. If we are to work towards this goal along the user action pathway, then we need communication trust. It helps to build effective relationships with those with whom we work and for whom we care. It connects us with one another.

- *Competence trust:* This is essentially a trust of capability. How far do you trust the people to whom you hand over? Do you trust them to do a good job? How far do you trust your patients/clients to give you an honest opinion about the quality of the care they are receiving, while still receiving it? How capable do you feel service users are in giving you constructive feedback? How capable are they in providing you with what you think you want and need to know, in order to continue to improve services? It used to be the norm that service users placed their trust in healthcare professionals. Recent high-profile cases that have caught the attention of the media have put competence trust under pressure. Now there is a discernable shift away from a 'trust me' attitude to a 'show me' attitude; in other words, away from placing our trust in character ('Trust me: I'm a doctor') and communication ('I will try to do my best') and towards competence trust ('This is my record in performing this particular surgical intervention').

A patient-led NHS beckons a hopeful and possible future. But it cannot be achieved alone. We cannot get there without communicating with and understanding each other. So it follows that we cannot build a reflective healthcare organisation without thinking deeply about two fundamental questions: What do I believe about others? What can I learn from others?

Building a language of positive regard through open listening

Kahane (2004) gives us a sharp reminder of the way some interactions inside healthcare organisations can go:

> The root of not listening is knowing. If I already know the truth, why do I need to listen to you? Perhaps out of politeness or guile I should pretend to listen, but what I really need to do is to tell you what I know, and if you don't listen, to tell you again, more forcefully. All authoritarian systems rest on the assumption that the boss can and does know the one right answer.

(Kahane 2004, p. 47)

Communication trust means talking openly and honestly. It brings with it a willingness, and ability on our part, to disclose to others what is in our head and heart. Listening openly, on the other hand, means being willing and able to positively embrace something different and new. This is not as easy as it may sound, because it involves issues about interpersonal relations, power, value alignment, and so on.

> My team worked hard to learn how to listen, without judging, to what another person was trying to say – really to be there. If we listen in the normal closed way, for what is right and what is wrong, then we won't be able to hear what is possible . . . We won't be able to create anything new.

(Kahane 2004, p. 77)

Listening sounds so simple. So I ask: When was the last time you felt you were listened to, openly? How far can you think of a positive experience, between you and a patient/client, when you felt you were listening openly to them? How do you know this? What made you feel this way? What were the circumstances that led up to this? What was the root cause of such a positive experience?

So what kinds of behaviour support the way we might openly listen to, and learn from, service users? How might this help us build a conversation between us of positive regard? Wheatley (2002, p. 28) offers us some useful thoughts in what she eloquently describes as 'seeing how wise we can be together'. What we can learn from Wheatley's work is that to make progress along this action pathway and to see this as enabling us to build a reflective healthcare organisation, we have to learn not only to listen openly but also to *listen reflectively*. Here are some of her thoughts:

- *We need to learn how to acknowledge one another as equals*: A language of positive regard requires us to acknowledge that we are equal as human beings (unequal when in role) and that we need each other. We cannot always improve services by trying to figure things out on our own.
- *We need to try to stay curious about each other*: We need to be genuinely interested in what service users have to say, not fearful. We need to test out our commitment to a value of the kind 'I believe that I can learn something significant from every patient/client I meet, each day' (Ghaye & Lillyman 2000). This weaves openness together with reflection.

- *We need to help each other listen openly and then act appropriately:* It can be hard work to listen, especially when we are busy, feeling certain of ourselves, or stressed. Try to think of a positive experience with your patients/clients when you know you listened to their views and then acted appropriately on them? What made this a positive experience?
- *We need to slow down to make time to listen reflectively:* If listening is an important part in developing a language of positive regard, so too is slowing down. Often we need to make time to listen to service users' views and to reflect on them.
- *We need to expect it to be messy at times:* Conversations, just like the building of a reflective organisation, do not move in a straight line. When learning from service users, it is probable that some things do not appear to connect with our experiences and perceptions. Experiences can be diverse. Listening openly and reflectively means that we resist the impulse to tidy things up and put experiences in little boxes. We need to learn the benefits of being 'disturbed'. By this, I mean having our ideas and practices challenged by others, by service users. How can we be creative in improving healthcare services if we are not willing to be disturbed?

To create new realities, we have to listen reflectively. It is not enough to be able to hear clearly the chorus of other voices; we must also hear the contribution of our own voice. It is not enough to be able to see others in the picture of what is going on; we must also see what we ourselves are doing. It is not enough to be observers of the problem situation; we must also recognise ourselves as actors who influence the outcome.

(Kahane 2004, p. 83)

Learning from service users: positive engagement

Earlier I referred to a maternity project supported by the Institute of Reflective Practice. The project was undertaken in a large urban area, over three years, and in partnership with a strategic health authority and a local supervising authority for midwives. A substantial number of women, as users of maternity services, were invited to help staff involved develop maternity services, so that they were more in line with what woman and their families felt they needed and wanted. The part of the project I refer to next was called 'Learning from You'. Box 3.3 shows a copy of the letter of invitation given to women accessing services in ten maternity units. The letter, and all the additional ways we learned from service users, had full ethics committee approval. Through this letter, we tried to convey the spirit of being valued, of listening and learning, and of positive regard that I have set out above. We asked if we could learn from women twice, over a period of 16 months. Data from the first invitation formed an initial benchmark. Data from the second invitation were compared with this benchmark. Benchmark 1 and 2 data were then fed back in a visually attractive, understandable graphical form. Without positive engagement, we do not stand a chance of harnessing the ingenuity

Box 3.3   Letter of invitation to learn from service user experiences

Dear Service User,

WOMEN'S EXPERIENCES OF MATERNITY SERVICES IN
xxxxxxxxxxxxx

You are invited to take part in a survey of maternity service users. Before you make any decisions it is important for you to understand why the survey is being undertaken and what it will involve. Please take the time to read the following information carefully and discuss it with others if you wish. *Take time to decide whether or not you want to take part.*

The survey is an important part of a project designed to develop maternity services so that they are more in line with what women and their families need and want. This survey aims to find out what experiences you had when using the service. *The results will be used to help improve maternity care.* You have been invited to take part because you have used maternity services in xxxxxxxxxx during xxxxxxxxxx. It is up to you to decide whether or not to take part. If you do consent, *fill in the enclosed questionnaire and return it.* To do this please:

- *Seal it* in the *white envelope* first.
- Then either *hand it to the person* giving you most of your xxxxxxxx care.
- Or *return it, by hand, to the clinic or ward* where this pack was given to you. Please put it in one of the 'Survey Boxes' there.
- Or *post it* in the enclosed white (pre-paid) envelope at any post box.

You may refuse to participate by not completing or returning the form. You do not need to give a reason for your decision and your care will not be affected in any way. The questionnaire normally takes 10 minutes to do. The information you supply will not be used to identify you. **Your name and any personal details will not be made public**.

If you wish to have further information about the survey, or would like help in completing the questionnaire, please speak to your midwife, or someone else in the maternity unit, who will arrange for someone to help you.

Thank you for taking part in this important work.

and creativity of service user knowledge necessary for developing even better services. With it, we begin to create a new kind of *blended system* for improvement – a blend of local and central, professional and service user interests and experiences, interacting both within and across all parts of the NHS. I look at this as a kind of 'adaptive challenge' (Heifetz & Linsky 2002). Positive engagement is not a new challenge, but it is still a difficult one to do well.

Two questionnaires were developed, piloted and validated. One covered antenatal care, the other labour and postnatal care. Each questionnaire was developed from an item bank of statements, offered to Institute staff, from women and men participating in three focus group meetings. All women participants already had one child. Attendance at these meetings was entirely voluntary. A total of 16 women and 5 men attended the 3 feedback sessions, each of 45 minutes duration, when they were collecting their child from a local playgroup. Through an iterative series (three cycles) of refinement after focus group feedback, each questionnaire was improved until it had high face and content validity. The drafts were then critically scrutinised by three experienced healthcare professionals, two of whom were heads of midwifery. Amendments were then discussed at two project board meetings. Further refinement of the content of each questionnaire and its administration followed as they were tested against Meleis' (1996) eight categories of human experience essential for culturally competent scholarship. These are:

- *Contextuality:* We learnt as much as we could from maternity staff about the participant's sociocultural and economic situation and had this in mind when framing the statements in each questionnaire.
- *Relevance:* The content of the questionnaires was drawn from actual statements offered to us from those who attended the focus group meetings. These were further enriched by the contents from a number of published papers (Department of Health 2003, 2004, Maternity Care Working Party 2006, NHS Modernisation Agency 2004).
- *Communication styles:* We were conscious that the languages we used were appropriate. The questionnaires were translated into seven different languages and a Braille version.
- *Awareness of identity and power differentials:* To try to address this, women were able to ask for help when completing the questionnaire. For some, this gave rise to a feeling of joint responsibility for its completion.
- *Disclosure:* Through written and verbal explanation and support from unit staff, every effort was made to build trust and secure authentic data from women.
- *Reciprocation:* This was about who gets what out of the survey. There had to be some gains for both parties, that is for us and the women who returned the questionnaires.
- *Empowerment:* Understandability, ease of questionnaire completion and return, and the right to not participate were goals, ensuring that women felt they were in control of the process.
- *Time:* We tried to be flexible in the use of time and extended the data-gathering window by four months in order to make sure that we were being as inclusive as possible.

Figure 3.4 shows an example of the antenatal questionnaire we used. We received 823 usable returns. This provided a secure database from which to build a positive action plan. The box on the back cover of the questionnaire was an open space for free writing.

FRONT PAGE

LEARNING FROM YOU

ANTENATAL CARE

PLEASE TICK A BOX

Is this your first baby?	I am	I am ....
Yes ☐	16–19 yrs ☐	White British ☐
No ☐	20–24 ☐	White Irish ☐
	25–29 ☐	Any other White background ☐
	30–34 ☐	Mixed white & black Caribbean ☐
	35–39 ☐	Mixed white and black African ☐
	40–44 ☐	Mixed white and Asian ☐
	Over 45 yrs ☐	Asian Indian ☐
		Asian Pakistani ☐
		Asian Bangladeshi ☐
		Any other Asian background ☐
		Black Caribbean ☐
		Black African ☐
		Any other Black background ☐
		Chinese ☐
		Other?...

© The Institute of Reflective Practice - UK

Figure 3.4   An example of an antenatal care questionnaire that was a catalyst for reflection, discussion and action.

ABOUT MY ANTENATAL CARE...

Please tick a box	GP	Midwife	Other Healthcare Professional	
1	The **first professional** I saw when I became pregnant was:				

		Less than 8 weeks	8–12 weeks	12–20 weeks	More than 20 weeks
2	When **I first saw** this professional my pregnancy was:				
3	When **I first met a midwife** my pregnancy was:				

		Yes by Midwife	Yes by GP	Yes by Other Healthcare Professional	No
4	I was given choices about **where to go** for my antenatal care				
5	I was given choices about **who would provide** my antenatal care				
6	I was given choices about **where I could** have my baby				

		Mostly Yes	Mostly No
7	I was given **information** about **staying healthy during** my pregnancy		
8	I felt my views were **listened to** and **acted upon**		
9	I could always **talk to staff** in private		

For office use only	A	C	PD	I	V

Figure 3.4 (Continued)

ABOUT MY ANTENATAL CARE...

	Please tick a box	Mostly Yes	Mostly No
10	I felt I **was** given **clear information** at the **right** time		
11	**I knew how** to **contact** a **named midwife** throughout my pregnancy		
12	Staff **always discussed** things with me		
13	Staff **understood** my **personal beliefs**		
14	**I could talk** to staff about my **real fears**		
15	I felt **involved** in **making decisions** about my pregnancy		
16	My **personal views** were **given respect**		
17	I felt well **prepared** for my **labour**		
18	I was **helped** to make my **own decisions** about my care		
19	Staff **respected** my **lifestyle**		
20	I felt **reassured** about the **best ways** to **prepare** for my baby		

PLEASE TURN OVER

Figure 3.4   (Continued)

BACK PAGE

Please tell us what you think

My experience would have been better if ......

(Write in this box)

Information about the project will be made widely available to you. Please contact xxxxxxxxxxxx if you wish to know more about this.

Contact: xxxxxxxxxxxxxxx

Email: xxxxxxxxxxxxxxxx

Write to: xxxxxxxxxxxxxx

© The Institute of Reflective Practice - UK

Figure 3.4   (Continued)

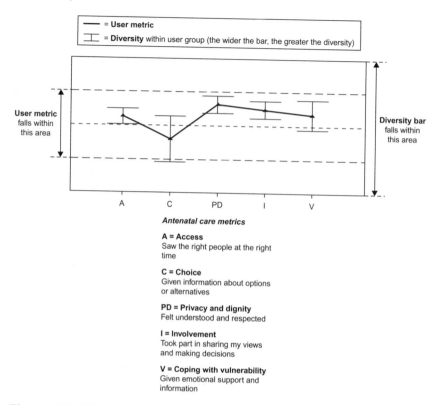

Figure 3.5   Fifty-three women's experiences of antenatal care in one maternity unit.

Figures 3.5–3.7 show some of the ways the results of the antenatal questionnaire were fed back. Statements were clustered around five metrics. A summary definition of each metric is provided. Figure 3.5 shows how a group of 53 women in one unit experienced antenatal care. The continuous line is the group norm. The bars represent the diversity of the women's experiences in relation to each metric; the wider the bar, the greater the diversity (or variation) of experience. Figure 3.6 illustrates how we fed back the results to enable women to productively engage in a conversation about the different experiences of women having their first and second or subsequent babies. Figure 3.7 shows a portrait that enabled those involved to reflect upon the significance of the relationship of age and their experience of antenatal care in a unit. Portraits depicting the experiences of women from specific ethnic groups were also fed back.

By utilising processes similar to those described above, we give ourselves a chance to scale up r-learning through this user action pathway. Critical to its success is building trust with service users, engaging positively with them, actively listening to what they have to say and then using the full power of feedback. Folkman (2006) says:

> Feedback can be very powerful. Those who look for and accept it position themselves to be more competent and capable. Those who resist, reject, or

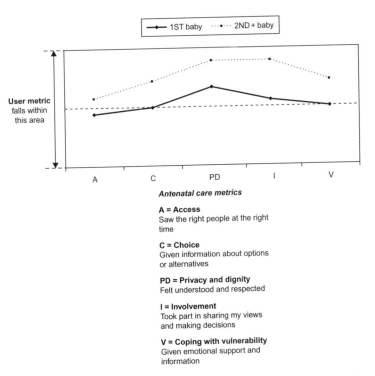

Figure 3.6 Experiences of 27 women having either their first or second/subsequent baby in a maternity unit.

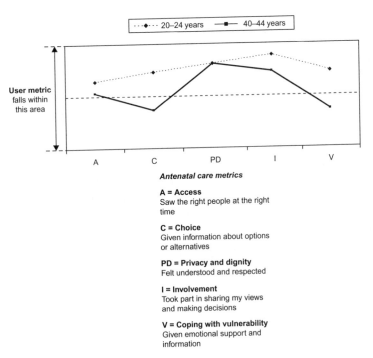

Figure 3.7 Relationship of age and antenatal experiences of 35 women in a maternity unit.

avoid it doom themselves to the limitations of their own personal insights, which may be right or wrong, but they will never know . . . Without feedback we are flying blind.

(Folkman 2006, p. xv)

Through appropriate feedback and reflection upon it, we have an opportunity to improve services through conversation.

Ideas for improvement

An additional resource generated by this process was service users' 'ideas for improvement'. We received 546 ideas in total, 114 from women and 432 from staff. There were repeats of the same idea, but through content analysis we derived 57 different ideas from women. These were organised into five 'ideas bundles' and fed back mainly (at the time of writing this book) through maternity service liaison committees and to staff groups. The bundles were called:

- 'care environment';
- 'quality of care';
- 'administration and information';
- 'visiting';
- 'food'.

Box 3.4 shows some of the ideas from the bundle 'quality of care'.

The language we use when feeding back information to service users is critical. Some languages 'welcome in', while some serve to 'exclude'. Some are more deficit-based, while some are more strengths-based. In building the reflective healthcare organisation through action pathways such as this, we need to develop good work habits that help us to move away from seeing feedback as 'helping us to sort out what's going wrong and then fixing it'. Part of the language of positive regard, as I characterise it, means that we do not regard organisational improvement as focusing on the negative and fixing all weaknesses. In the work of Folkman (2006), we find evidence that the key to predicting success is not the absence of weaknesses but rather the presence of a few profound strengths. He argues that one crucial role of feedback is to enable people and organisations to better understand the skills and processes that could be developed into profound strengths.

A key to being highly successful is doing some things well. Investing all our time and energy in fixing our weaknesses does not necessarily help us build strengths.

(Folkman 2006, p. xix)

Box 3.4 Some ideas from women about how their experiences of maternity services might have been improved further

- Growth scan should be routinely offered in the third trimester.
- An obstetrician could be seen as part of regular care, especially if there are any concerns, rather than having to ask directly to see one.
- I could have met the midwife who would be delivering my baby. At 38 weeks I feel like I have met everyone but the midwives on the labour ward.
- I needed to be given a more experienced midwife who actually listens to what you're saying and feeling, as I am a prima gravida, so everything's a new experience for me.
- Seeing the same midwife at every visit.
- Domino system of midwife maternity care (available elsewhere in the UK) would be very attractive.
- In the early stages of pregnancy (i.e. between 12-week scan and 28-week midwife appointment), the schedule of care needs to be more clear and more frequent.
- All staff on all wards need to be more caring. On the ward I was on, staff were cursory, quick to judge about right and wrong, and with little time or desire.
- A consultant one hasn't met would introduce themselves. It's hard to know who does what.
- People could have been a little more polite. I felt un-respected and some people were so rude. Every time I asked about something, they just bit my head off.
- If we can't get a specific midwife to look after us, then we need to feel confident that different midwives can be consistent.
- I would have felt better if someone had read the previous notes and I had one person or midwife to talk through my history with.
- I could have been routinely offered a follow-up visit at my home, say three weeks after delivery to discuss feeding, etc.
- More night staff.

I suggest that the act of inviting feedback tends to increase others' expectations that we will change and improve services in some positive way. To build a reflective organisation means that we need to learn to sustain positive feedback processes – processes that discourage reactions such as 'That's terrible' and encourage other reactions such as 'That's interesting' or 'That's useful' and even 'I understand how we can use this positively'.

Building a reflective organisation means that we need to sustain conversations of positive regard with service users through:

- trust
- engagement
- open and reflective listening
- feedback.

Progress along this action pathway requires us to ask the reflective questions 'What can I learn from service users' experience?' and 'How can learning from users of services become an organisation-wide work habit?'

Action pathway: leadership

In an article in the *Health Service Journal*, Carlisle writes:

> Last week the prime minister [Tony Blair] announced a new scheme to bring the experience of people leading FTSE100 companies into the NHS. It's not the first time this and other governments have tried to harness commercial acumen and leadership skills from industry and other parts of the public sector to develop the management of the health service. Beneath all this lies a simple question: What makes a good leader? And this sparks further impossible debate. Does the NHS set its leaders an impossible challenge? What could the health service learn from leaders in other industries? Do the low levels of recruitment from sectors outside the health service reflect the complex challenge of running NHS organisations or an entrenched cultural resistance to outsiders?

(Carlisle 2006, p. 34)

In this section I take up the challenge of learning from the experiences of leadership on the 'outside'. Maybe we need to learn to 'de-centre' more often, take a good look at the reasons for the existence of any 'cultural resistance' and see what comes into view when we reflect on leadership challenges from an 'outside looking in' perspective. This is different from always seeing the world from within the fishbowl. The NHS Institute for Innovation and Improvement is doing much good work in learning what it can from manufacturing and service industries and then applying this to the management of healthcare delivery. One example of this is its best-practice project initiative called the 'productive series' (Bevan 2006). The first was launched in April 2007 and is called 'The Productive Ward'; this will be followed by 'The Productive Community Hospital'. Even so, there is still much more learning to be done.

In Table 0.3 I summarised some of the attributes that determine the complexity and duration of action along each pathway-to-scale. Here I discuss two important aspects of building a reflective healthcare organisation through the leadership pathway. Both link with my earlier discussion about *appreciation* and *tipping*. One is concerned with leadership and appreciative intelligence; the other is about tipping-point leadership.

Leadership through appreciative intelligence

The 'must read' for all those interested in appreciative intelligence and the way it can be applied judiciously to building a reflective healthcare organisation is Thatchenkery & Metzker (2006). In a nutshell, appreciative intelligence (or PN, as I shall now call it) is about our ability to re-frame a given situation and, in so doing, to recognise the positive possibilities embedded in it, but not necessarily apparent to the untrained eye. PN also involves action – the necessary action to positively engage with others so that valued outcomes unfold from the generative aspects of the current situation. PN is situated in the field of multiple intelligences, something proposed by Howard Gardner (1993) in his book *Frames of Mind: The Theory of Multiple Intelligences*. Gardner demonstrated that intelligence was not a single ability but a number of capacities. He based his view on findings from disciplines such as anthropology, psychology and cognitive science and from the biographies of exceptional individuals. Thatchenkery & Metzker (2006) argue that PN is another type of intelligence within the multiple intelligence field.

Three components of appreciative intelligence

Thatchenkery & Metzker (2006) propose that there are three components of PN: the ability to re-frame, appreciate the positive and see how the future unfolds from the present. For this to happen, we need to be persistent, have self-belief, have a tolerance for uncertainty and have irrepressible resilience.

> Because the people we interviewed could reframe, appreciate the positive and see how the future could unfold from the present, they could see how their end goal was possible to accomplish. Thus, they were willing to persist and to believe that their own actions and abilities would take them to a successful conclusion. Because they could envision the way a positive future could unfold from the present, they could deal with the uncertainty that often accompanies a new venture . . . or a crisis. They exhibited irrepressible resilience, the ability to bounce back from a difficult situation, as the result of reframing, seeing what was positive in the situation, and understanding that a better future could come about despite a crisis or setback.

(Thatchenkery & Metzker 2006, pp. 15–16)

These three basic components of PN are very much in evidence in the way I have tried to re-frame reflective practice as r-learning and, in doing so, bring the field into some kind of wholeness (see Figure 0.2). Re-framing is not just about seeing things differently; it is also about choice. When we choose to pay attention to one aspect of a clinical encounter, for the time being we are choosing to ignore other aspects of it. What we attend to is usually related to our values, in the sense that focusing on something implies that we value it. What we choose to ignore is, in some way, less important, less valuable or less interesting right now. *Appreciating the positive* refers to the processes of selectivity and judgement of some person or thing's value or worth. When meeting those who work in health and social care for the first time, Institute of Reflective Practice staff usually try to create a space for an 'appreciative pairs' activity. In essence, this is about trying to see the best in people, their unique gifts, talents and qualities.

Appreciative pair work

Appreciative pair working is described in a paper I co-wrote with Anita Melander-Wikman and Maria Jansson, both from Luleå University of Technology, Sweden. We called the paper 'Reflections on an appreciative approach to empowering elderly people, in home healthcare' (Melander-Wikman *et al.* 2006). The paper was a reflective account of aspects of our collective interest in developing and sustaining ways that might enable elderly people to feel more empowered to exercise their right of self-determination. The context was that of home healthcare in northern Sweden. The living data for this paper were drawn from two days of workshop activities with 35 homecare staff working in the municipality of Luleå, Sweden. The workshop was one outcome of the e-Home Health Care @ North Calotte (eHHC) Project of 2003–05. We concluded the paper with some collective reflections about (i) the *practices* of participation (e.g. dialogue) and an *intention* of it (e.g. empowerment) in the context of valuing elderly clients' involvement in accelerating service change; (ii) how to re-frame traditional views of the relationships between research and practice and, as a consequence, open up new possibilities for understanding how elderly people's lived experiences can be a positive force for service improvement; and (iii) the use of storyboards as an appreciative approach to enable frontline staff to reflect on their work, share and learn together.

Establishing an appreciative disposition

At the start of each day's workshop, we invited homecare staff, some of whom knew each other well, to engage in two activities in order to acknowledge that an appreciative disposition towards each other, their clients and their service, would be needed throughout the day. The three of us, as facilitators, had known each other for four years. Anita Melander-Wikman's field is physiotherapy, Maria Jansson's is information systems and mine is educare. We began in a circle inviting homecare staff to form pairs. We joined in this activity as well. Our invitation was:

> Spend five minutes discovering something of the best about your partner. Use the time you have to discover something you most appreciate or admire in them. We will then be inviting you to share this appreciation with others in the room. So please check out with your partner how far they are OK with what you will say.

This activity was a way of trying to positively frame the whole day. It was a way of (re-)grounding relationships (Chaffee 2005). What was shared was astonishing, powerful, insightful, believable and humorous.

One woman said: 'I've been working with Sonia for ten years and I still can't find anything positive to say about her!' When the slightly nervous laughter died down, she said: 'Seriously, I want to say that Sonia can do things that I can only dream about. She is sensitive, creative and very good at her work.'

Appreciative circles

The second activity was even more interactive. All staff had to work together to achieve success. Eight string circles, of different sizes, were laid on to the floor. Our invitation was: 'When I say "Now", please choose a circle and go and stand inside it, making sure both feet are inside the circle.' For the first two rounds, there was more circle space than was needed for staff. They were spoilt for choice. Then for the next seven rounds, the instruction was the same, but one string circle was taken away each time. As choice diminished, homecare staff had to make key decisions about where they were going to stand and with whom. They had to be creative in the way they made sure both feet were inside the circle. When there was only one string circle left the instruction was: 'Now there is no more choice. Come together here, making sure both of your feet are inside the circle.' Some rushed into doing what they had done before. But they soon appreciated that they had to act differently if they were to achieve the task. They had to listen carefully to what was said. There simply was not sufficient room inside the circle for doing things the same way. Creative discussion, active listening, trial and error, and partnerships were all in evidence. When they achieved the goal, there was spontaneous applause, a valuing of a job well done.

Working from the 'positive present'

The third component of PN is seeing how the future unfolds from the present.

> The implication of the second component is that useful, desirable, or positive aspects already exist in the current condition of people, situations or things, but sometimes they must be revealed, unlocked, or realised. People with high appreciative intelligence connect the generative aspects of the present with a desirable end goal. They see how the future unfolds from the present ... Many people have the ability to reframe and the capacity to appreciate the positive. Yet, if they don't see the concrete ways that the possibilities of the present moment could be channelled, they have not developed appreciative intelligence.

(Thatchenkery & Metzker 2006, p. 7)

Often, this third component is a real stumbling block. It involves everyone at least drawing a distinction between what they feel they can do themselves and what they can do with help and support from others.

In our work in home healthcare, we built on appreciative pair and circle work by encouraging homecare staff to reflect upon their own practice. We

Table 3.1   Some reflections on practice by homecare staff.

Something I feel I can *improve* in my work (blue sheets)	Something I feel I am very *good* at in my work (yellow sheets)
Stop putting up boundaries in my work and not take over others' responsibility	Listening to my colleagues
Listen to myself and trust my own judgement	Listening to people having a hard time
Delegate more	Listen! Reach out to people
Structure my work better	Empathy
Try to keep better documentation	Create a good atmosphere and be encouraging
I'm not sure	Organising my work
Express myself better	Finding solutions to problems
Be able to handle conflict better	Planning and structuring
Not trust people too much	Don't know
Give feedback	I have patience in my work
Be able to plan for better cooperation between different professionals	Able to stay calm in different situations

provided them with two coloured pieces of paper. On the blue paper we asked staff to write down how they thought they might improve one aspect of their work. On the yellow paper, we asked them to state something that they felt they were very good at in their daily work. We encouraged them to forget being modest! In groups of four to five people, they then discussed what they had written on all the pieces of paper. Each small group then brought one blue and one yellow piece of paper to the front, something their group thought was significant to them, and presented this to others. Table 3.1 sets out some of their responses. When each group had presented, we were able to ask the question 'Do any common themes emerge from these reflections?' This produced considerable discussion.

So what did the three of us appreciate from undertaking these activities?

Anita: Working together with people, both clients and staff, seems to demand but also create energy. It is important to create a culture at work that helps in this balance so that staff, in their ambitions to create good homecare services, will not be drained of energy. I learnt that if you listen and learn from others, from what they are good at, this can help you create a positive strategy at work.

Maria: I learnt that we are very good at talking about what we like to improve but not so good at talking about what we are really good at. Therefore, it is important that we can have workshops like this, appreciating each other's knowledge and learning from each other.

Tony: I learnt that we need to develop reflective activities that are uncomplicated and enjoyable for frontline staff to engage with. Activities that are inclusive, participatory and as non-threatening as possible, that don't take too much time to do but that have the potential for high yield. In other words, through dialogue, we amplify not only what concerns us but also what creates energy and joy in our daily work.

Leading through appreciation

In Stavros & Torres (2005), we begin to get a feel for the potential of a creative synthesis of PN and leadership. What I call 'leading though appreciation' is an important part of r-learning because, fundamentally, it requires both reflection and action. In general, I suggest that leading through appreciation requires:

- leaders to use their appreciative intelligence;
- leaders to understand the positive dynamics that contribute to the quality of their working relationships with others. Part of this are a willingness and ability to get to the root causes of:
  - what's working well;
  - what gives life and provides positive energy to working relationships, particularly when staff feel they are working under pressure;
  - how we come to be successful, meet targets and service user needs;
  - how we establish our positive core (see action step 4, p. 220).

Stavros & Torres (2005) present some important reflective questions that help orient us to the notion of leading through appreciation. One reading of these questions is that they encourage us to consider alternatives. The questions are:

- How are we responding or reacting to one another?
- What are we aware of (assumptions, beliefs, thoughts, feelings, etc.)?
- What are we working to create, and how are we creating meaning together?

Their hope is that these questions might lead us to respond to further reflective questions such as:

- How did I come to understand things the way I do, when it seems so different from you?
- How can we come to understand one another and create shared meaning?
- What meaning will my actions have for others?
- How are my actions influencing relationships here?

(Stavros & Torres 2005, p. 25)

The need for a spirit of enquiry

Throughout this book I have tried to argue that a focus on deficiencies, root cause analysis, remedial action planning, closing gaps, deficit-based conversations, putting lots of energy into interventions in clogged-up and broken-down systems, machine metaphors (Morgan 2006), and so on are still are among the most recognisable and audible vocabularies in many healthcare organisations. I have implied that these approaches may well have reached their point of diminishing return. There is an increasing amount of collective wisdom that leads us to believe that this is the case, especially in flatter, more responsive, empowered and team-based healthcare organisations. Additionally, I have suggested that in order to build a different kind of organisational mindscape – a reflective one – and to reap the benefits of this, we need the courage to think and act differently. In a book by Schiller *et al.* (2001), we find a compelling argument for a concept of leadership as a process of reality construction and meaning-making, not leadership as machine repair. Central to this conception is a *spirit of enquiry*, which, Schiller *et al.* say, is even more powerful in leadership than final answers and interventions. They stress that organisations are centres of human-relatedness first and foremost, and relationships thrive where there is an appreciative eye and when people see the best in one another. When positively affirming work patterns enable everyone to have a voice and be heard, they argue that possibilities are created not only for new services but for better services, not new structures and organisations but better structures and organisations.

So what are some of the actions of those leading through appreciation? Here are some suggestions:

- Lead by valuing, not evaluating.
- Create change by synthesising and combining capabilities, not just fixing the problematic.
- Imagine the new, the better and the possible in ways that energise, uplift and bring others on board.
- Create an alignment of values and strengths that help to make people's weaknesses less consuming.
- Magnify all that is good and best in people.
- Define, nourish and communicate to everyone the organisation's positive core.
- Sustain conversations of positive regard.
- Try to enlarge everyone's knowledge, skills and vision.
- Continuously try to expand the web of inclusion, enabling individuals and teams to respond to diversity positively.

Tipping-point leadership

In the action pathway-to-scale that I called 'conversation', I summarised the idea of the tipping point and how it has its roots in epidemiology. An understanding of the tipping point is crucial if we are to see how the future (the reflective healthcare organisation) unfolds from the present. Here I want to apply the notion to leadership. We cannot get the process of scaling up r-learning to tip towards a systemic work habit unless we take seriously the column in Table 0.3 that refers to the concept of 'critical mass'. For the process to tip, an organisation needs leaders who can make an unforgettable and compelling case for r-learning. Framing this challenge is critical. It is a subtle and sensitive task. The goal needs to be perceived as achievable, as attainable. If scaling up r-learning is perceived as mission impossible, then it will not happen. If there have been some successes with r-learning, for example with individuals or clinical teams, no matter how small, then the challenge might be framed as successes to be repeated or enlarged. Additionally, these people need to concentrate what resources they have and to scale up r-learning on what matters most. They also need to mobilise the commitment of the organisation's key players and power brokers, and do all this with an appreciative eye. This is quite a challenge, especially if we find ourselves working in an organisation where a significant number of healthcare staff are wedded to preserving the status quo, for whatever reasons, and especially if staff feel demoralised, demotivated, disaffected, tired or anxious. This was brought home to me when I met a multidisciplinary team from an acute trust for a day set up by the organisation. The day was called 'Better teams – better care'. As the first three individuals entered the room, I was greeted with 'Is this going to be any good then?', followed by 'I'm tired' and 'Do I have to be here?' You might perceive this as not the most positive of beginnings. But if we re-frame things, the three comments were invaluable. The first became a challenge: 'So let's see if we can make it a worthwhile day and to do this we might have to try to give the day a chance'. The other two comments reminded me that at some point during the day I needed to explore, with everyone, those times at work when they were not so tired and did not feel coerced into doing something that they did not want to do. From this, we then needed to ask questions about the root causes of such positive feelings and how we might amplify them.

Can tipping-point leadership be learned?

Kim & Mauborgne (2003) argue that tipping-point leadership can be learned. Interestingly, they use a racecourse metaphor – hurdles and fences to be jumped, knocked over and broken through – to illustrate how we can overcome the forces of inertia and reach one or more tipping points. Their paper uses a deficit vocabulary. I have flipped this over and used a more strengths-based one. The essence of their paper is interpreted in this way:

- *Breaking through the cognitive hurdle:* This involves trying to get staff to agree to think about the root causes of past and current successes and the need to amplify these. It also involves getting staff to think of success as something they actually experience, not something they hear about happening to others. Communicating this in a clear and persuasive way means that the idea of success sticks with staff. Stickiness can be increased if leaders assert the moral purposes of r-learning, re-state its intentions, build capacity to scale it up, pay attention to the way values are (mis)aligned and keep success front and central in people's minds.

- *Sidestepping the resources hurdle:* Once staff engage in conversations about how the future unfolds from the positive present, they usually ask questions about resourcing this. A positive question is: 'How can an organisation tip without extra resources?' Obvious strategies are to concentrate on the people (e.g. clinical team) and in the places (e.g. a unit, department, community setting) where there has been the greatest success in breaking through the cognitive hurdle. Some of the biggest payoffs have the smallest impact on budgets, as I describe in some detail later. Acts that make staff feel more valued and respected often cost nothing.

- *Jumping the motivational hurdle:* Breaking through and sidestepping the first two hurdles is a good start. But if we are to scale up r-learning in the way I suggest, and reach a tipping point, then everyone in the organisation needs more than a knowledge of what needs to be done. They must also want it to happen. It is about getting a critical mass of staff sufficiently motivated to contribute to the scaling-up process. To do this, we need to harness the powers of the organisation's key language and people influencers. Additionally, an understanding of the generic processes of innovation (see p. 92) is important, especially the point about relative advantage (see p. 98).

- *Knocking over the political hurdle:* Any improvement process is a political one, because improvement is fundamentally about who gets what, where, how and why. Even if an organisation has reached a tipping point, powerful vested interests may still drag staff back into deficit-based conversations and remedial actions. Sometimes the closer we get to tipping, the more fiercely vocal the 'fixers' become. Tipping-point leaders use their appreciative intelligence (their persistence, conviction, tolerance and irrepressible resilience) to build appreciative allies and coalitions. They:

. . . reframe or reinterpret a given situation . . . to perceive that a positive consequence [can] be built from even the most drastic or devastating circumstances. Rather than experiencing a position of impossibility, and therefore a situation without hope or remedy, intelligent leaders [show] a capacity to see what is possible and to set a plan of action, with concrete steps to create the envisioned positive state.

(Thatchenkery & Metzker 2006, p. 29)

Building a reflective organisation means that we need to develop a critical mass of staff:

- with tipping-point leadership skills;
- who can exercise leadership with an appreciative eye;
- who can establish and sustain an appreciative disposition across the organisation;
- who work from the positive present.

Progress along this action pathway requires us to ask the reflective question: How can we have more staff who can lead through appreciation?

Action pathway: team

The central question in my book *Developing the Reflective Healthcare Team* (Ghaye 2005) is 'How can we develop reflective healthcare teams that are able to sustain high-quality, personalised care?' In this book, the central question reads: 'How can we scale up reflective learning so that it becomes an organisation-wide, sustainable work habit?' The difference between these two questions is that now I am inviting whole organisations (whole systems) to engage in r-learning, for the reasons I outlined in action step 1. As I explained earlier, scaling up is not simply a matter of creating more and more reflective teams. This is certainly a significant part, but it is not everything. Scaling up has to be understood through a multidisciplinary lens and with at least a working knowledge of innovation theory, decision, learning, activity and dynamic systems theories. In turn, this has to be supported with insights from social and organisational psychology and sociology. In practice, scaling up needs to be undertaken with courage, ethically and with a sense of moral purpose.

Learning from developing reflective teams

Previously I was critical of the conventional models that describe team development as a linear, step-by-step, sequential, one-way process (Ghaye 2005). A classic example of this is Tuckman's (1965) four-stage model, which includes forming, storming, norming and performing stages. Another traditional approach is one where development is associated with team roles (Belbin 1982). The work of Kur (1996), and his use of 'face' as a metaphor for team development, adds a different perspective. The basic idea behind Kur's work is that of teams having 'faces'. At one time a team may wear one face, and at another time the team may wear a different face. Each face is associated with certain patterns of relationships and action. The pattern is not linear but more complex. Any face may precede or follow any other face. Teams might move back and forth, presenting and then discarding faces according to the exigencies of the moment. Kur describes a total of five faces. At first glance they look remarkably similar to Tuckman's stages, but it is Kur's interpretation of the faces that is interesting. For example, his description of a team's *informing face* goes like this. When teams wear an informing face

> ... their members strive to understand, learn, evaluate and develop a shared mindset ... Informing is about coming to grips with shared values ... some teams do not engage in these learning processes until well into the life of the team, if at all.

(Kur 1996, p. 26)

Healthy teams need to embrace and return to their informing face from time to time. The different demands of working life may require this. In strengthening teams for high performance, Kur argues that we should try to develop conditions to enable teams to wear their *performing face* as frequently and as continuously as possible. Kur describes a team's performing face in terms of high trust, esprit, openness with one another, role flexibility, active listening and actively seeking ideas from each other. Additionally, decision-making is shared and '. . . any member of the team may act on behalf of the entire team in the confidence that his or her team-mates will support any action taken' (Kur 1996, p. 26). A team needing or wanting to change its face is a liberating way to view team development. Changing faces, in any direction, needs to be accepted as normal and responsive to the different demands of practice. Embracing r-learning enables us to do this sensitively and effectively. What is also helpful is the Robertson Cooper Ltd (2006) 'Teamable: making your teamwork' process. 'Teamable' is premised on a view that we all have a certain amount of flexibility around our typical ways of contributing to a team.

Direction of travel

I suggest that we need to be cautious of linear thinking, in any direction, when trying to build a reflective healthcare organisation. This is why I have drawn upon the metaphors of a 'journey' (van de Ven *et al.* 1999) and over 'rough ground' (Blair 2006) in this book. In reality, there is more than one trajectory (Miller 1990) or direction any healthcare team or organisation might travel. Evidence for this can be found in the former performance rating system for NHS trusts in England. Star ratings were produced and published by the Commission for Health Improvement (CHI), which was the independent regulator of NHS performance. The UK government was responsible for setting priorities, which in turn determined the indicators relating to key targets. Other indicators were designed by the CHI and the Department of Health to reflect a range of performance issues, following consultation with the service and other stakeholders. Trusts with the highest levels of performance are awarded a performance rating of three stars. Trusts with the poorest levels of performance against the indicators, or that had made little progress in implementing clinical governance arrangements, were awarded a performance rating of zero stars.

Between years, some trusts gained and others lost stars. These ratings were never designed to give a comprehensive picture of every aspect of the performance of NHS organisations. Nevertheless, the system was criticised heavily. For example:

> Performance indicators that 'name and shame' NHS organisations or individuals should be scrapped because they 'demoralise and antagonise' staff and damage the health service as a whole, the Royal Statistical Society said in a report released last week. The society says that public sector employees and the public are suspicious of government performance statistics and see them as being used

to meet political ends and as likely to be misreported by the media. The society wants the government to take a 'much wider consideration of the ethics and cost-effectiveness of performance monitoring' and to look at alternatives.

(Gould 2003, p. 1008)

From 2005, the Healthcare Commission introduced a far more wide-ranging system than that of star ratings called an 'annual health check'. The process scores NHS trusts on many aspects of performance, including the quality of the services the trust provides to patients and the public and how well the trust manages its finances and other resources, such as property and staff. Scores are based on a range of information gathered throughout the year.

From success to failure

What we have learned from team development gives us some insight into organisational development. For example, an organisation can take more than one route, or action pathway, to improving services and working lives. But just as with teams, when the heat is on, with targets that need to be met and a system that is cash-strapped and under pressure, there are some trajectories that lead, unfortunately, *from success to failure*. I caricature them thus:

- *Focusing trajectory:* Highly skilled, experienced professionals and support staff, committed to high-quality service provision, become inward-looking and target-obsessed. By focusing on details, they lose sight of the bigger picture.
- *Venturing trajectory:* Imaginative staff, who work together to build innovative, influential boundary-crossing teams, turn jealous guardians of resources and turf, not daring to venture into other worlds of (apparent) chaos, where new opportunities may be found.
- *Inventing trajectory:* Staff who value and promote a culture of questioning, who willingly and appreciatively accept ideas from everywhere, and who thrive on diversity, are accused of being out of touch, of losing the plot, of failing to 'get real' and of 'airy-fairy thinking'.
- *Decoupling trajectory:* Staff who take partnership working and service user participation seriously, and who cleverly add value to what they can by working with others in new ways, turn into escape-committee chairpersons, protecting their backs, and retreat into boxes because that is the last place left to them where they feel some sense of security and personal worth.

Different questions, different conversations

There is more to learn from trying to develop reflective teams. It is about understanding how staff inertia works and thus the way it might affect the scaling up of r-learning. I draw your attention to a number of common aspects of this. Much of the way inertia in organisations is described uses the deficit vocabularies I explained earlier. Maybe that is why inertia is always seen as a 'problem'. Some aspects, couched in a deficit-based rather than a strengths-based way, are:

- *Passivity:* Not acting in situations that need action. This includes doing nothing, uncritically accepting goals and suggestions made by others, becoming paralysed to act, or even becoming aggressive (shutting down or letting off steam).
- *Learned helplessness:* This helplessness means staff feel they can do nothing to change or improve the situation. There are degrees of helplessness, from statements such as 'I'm not up to this' to feelings of deep inadequacy often coupled with a depressive state. Staff feel that service improvement is not in their control, is outside of their sphere of influence and is not within their immediate experience.
- *Disabling self-talk:* This is where staff talk themselves out of things and into passivity. Conversations slide into an obsession with problems and obstacles. The vocabulary used is 'It won't work' and 'We can't do it.'
- *Vicious (not virtuous) cycles:* Plans do not go well. The future does not unfold from the present in the expected way. Staff feel knocked back. They begin to feel they are losing a sense of self-worth. They lose heart and confidence in their plan for change. This spirals staff downwards into a mindset of defeat and depression.
- *Feeling that things are falling apart:* Sometimes staff have a tendency to give up on action they have initiated. Action to implement a positive plan for change can begin strongly but then dwindle and stop. Plans seem realistic and achievable and begin with enthusiasm; then implementation becomes tedious. What seemed easy at the start now seems to be quite difficult. Staff flounder. They get discouraged and may give up.
- *Choosing not to change:* Some staff develop new understandings and awareness of themselves, others, their work and their workplace. They even appreciate what they need to do in order to change the current situation. But they choose not to act. They do not want to 'pay the price' called for by committing fully to the action.

Looking at things in another way

Let us look at this collection of 'problems' another way. Figure 0.2 showed us that the intentions of r-learning are to develop appreciations, re-frame experience, build collective wisdom, achieve and move forward. One way to re-frame inertia is to see it as staff being 'stuck'. A way to try to get 'unstuck' is to open up possibilities for different kinds of conversation, using more strengths-based vocabularies. One way I get staff to appreciate how different questions can generate different conversations is shown in Table 3.2. Usually I invite staff to organise themselves into two groups. Each group sits in a different part of the room. One group gets the four questions on the left-hand side of Table 3.2. The other group receives the

Table 3.2   Different questions, different conversations.

Deficit-based questions	Strengths-based questions
1 Think of a problem that you tackled at work this week Response:	1 Think of a success that you achieved at work this week Response:
2 What were the causes of the problem? Response:	2 What contributed to the success? Response:
3 What needs to stop in order to 'fix' the problem? Response:	3 What do you need to keep doing to create further success? Response:
4 What is one behaviour you will need to change, and how far can you do it? Response:	4 What is one behaviour you need to keep, and how will you keep doing it? Response:

strengths-based ones. Staff are asked not to talk aloud about the questions. Although they are generally curious about being in two groups, they often assume they are responding to the same questions. This is fine to begin with. They write individually. Then I invite 'deficit' group members to read aloud their responses to question 1. I also ask them what it felt like to do this task. After this, I turn to the other group. This time they read their responses to their question 1. I ask them the same question: What did it feel like to do this task? In these two acts, a *space* is created for some important learning to take place – learning about the way different questions generate different kinds of conversation. After acknowledging that each group has done something different, I mix up the groups. I invite staff to work in pairs and read though their responses to their deficit- or strengths-based questions. In conclusion I ask each pair to say what they feel they have learned so that we can collectively deepen our appreciation of the way we can build a more positive future.

Accelerating progress along this action pathway may depend upon the sustained use of the 'four practices of open space' (Owen 1997). In summary, these are:

- *Opening:* This is about opening hearts, creating opportunities to really listen to and learn from staff and user experiences, a willingness to be open to the possibility that 'we' don't always know best.
- *Inviting:* This is about inviting connection and creating spaces to explore how the future might positively unfold from the present.

- *Holding:* This is about supporting collaboration, working together to support desirable change and improvement, and providing space and time to engage in r-learning.
- *Practice:* This is about making a difference, moving from rhetoric to action, seeing things through, sustaining, realising and making talk of better services real. What is crucial in this practice is that those who can, acknowledge and reward those who are working towards building a better service.

Creating 'have moments'

A meeting with a large multidisciplinary group of staff working in maternity services was dominated by capacity and staffing problems. Everyone was well practised in their use of problem talk. After 30 minutes, staff began to look weary. This was a moment to try to see service delivery differently. I had worked with them before. At some point during each of these meetings, staff talked about one or all of these things: *not* feeling appreciated and respected, *not* coping well at work, and the fact that different ways of doing things were *not* valued in their clinical area. I asked them to get into three groups. I then invited each group to respond to one of these statements:

- Think about a really positive experience for you when you felt *appreciated and respected* at work.
- Think about a really positive experience for you when you felt you *were able to cope well with your work* here.
- Think about a really positive experience for you when you felt *different ways of doing things were valued* here.

A nursery nurse said 'I've never been asked this before.' A supervisor of midwives said 'This is a very different kind of question to answer than the usual ones.' The general manager said, revealingly, 'This is hard!' In Box 3.5 I include some of the responses to the first statement about appreciation and respect. In doing this, I wanted staff to experience what Adler & Fagley (2005) call a 'have moment'; in other words, to pay attention to what they have experienced and enjoyed rather than what they have not. I wanted them to stop, reflect and take notice of what was positive in their working lives. This takes a particular kind of disciplined thinking (Collins 2001). Their responses to the three statements provided us with a vocabulary to try to build a more positive future from the present.

Nurturing collective wisdom

Nurturing collective wisdom is a prerequisite for wise collective action. It is through r-learning activities like the ones suggested here that we unlock and can cultivate the intellectual and moral resources and commitment of staff in order to improve services and their working lives. This process is what Surowiecki (2004) calls 'accessing the wisdom of crowds'. Surowiecki suggests four key conditions for collective wisdom to function well:

Box 3.5 Some staff responses to a 'have moment'

Question: 'Think about a really positive experience for you when you felt *appreciated* and *respected* at work'

- After one very hectic, stressful night, a colleague came on duty and right away, without asking, made cups of tea.
- When as midwives, nursery nurses and HCAs we help each other to look after and carry out work even if we are not allocated to the patient. The midwife working with me was very appreciative and thanked me for being a good team player.
- Despite the ward being extremely busy, when the staff work together and thank you for giving your assistance. This makes me feel appreciated and respected, so you don't mind the hard work.
- Having a busy and frustrating day, not knowing if the woman would get better or worse. Then getting told 'Thank you. You have been a great help.'
- To be thanked by a patient who I cared for over a six-month period on the ward and still get thank-you cards occasionally ten years after.
- If I am ever late for duty, I am always greeted and welcomed on arrival.
- I spent time assisting a woman to breastfeed her baby. Her response and thanks made me feel glad that I had taken the time to do so.
- Happy when the women have had a lovely delivery. We all got to know each other.
- When I helped the nursery nurses to bath and feed the babies and they showed their appreciation for my efforts. Sitting with colleagues having a lovely cup of tea together.
- A new mum with a baby boy was very frustrated. She couldn't settle her baby. I came into her room and asked if she wanted to talk to anybody who could help her stop her baby crying. Then I started talking to her and winding the baby, who did a huge burp and I showed her how to do it. At the end of my shift, I came back to see her and she said thank you.
- The doctors appreciating your contribution to care.
- When you receive thanks from a patient, for example a thank-you card, gift, etc. You feel appreciated and touched with the time they have taken to write it or thought of that gift or a general verbal thank-you.
- A lady spent five days on the ward when I first started. Her baby was small and mum's first child. She wrote me a letter and was pleased to have met me at that time.
- Helping a patient to establish breastfeeding following a mastectomy.

- People need to feel *independent* of one another, to feel their opinions are not determined by those around them.
- People need to be *diverse* enough to represent a range of backgrounds, needs and interests.
- People need to be sufficiently *decentralised*, whereby they are able to specialise and draw on their local knowledge.
- There has to be some means, either formal or informal, for *aggregation*; in other words, to turn independent views and judgements into collective wisdom.

From model to appreciative framework

Ghaye (2005) culminated in the presentation of what I called 'a generic and holistic framework for developing the reflective healthcare team'. It was based on 'the wisdom of the crowds' that comprised 753 teams of health and social care staff and 3211 service user experiences in the UK between 1999 and 2004. The key features and processes of the framework were the following:

- It *focused on team learning*, facilitated through the interests and practices of reflection. It linked team development with the team's ability to learn. It made *learning and development visible* to all those involved.
- It was underpinned by forms of *disciplined and supported reflection and action*, which enabled teams to sustain high-quality personalised care.
- It *emphasised learning through sharing*. This process influences a team's wellness and general health. Wellness affects how far a team is able to influence change and respond positively to it.
- It viewed the development of reflective teams as a social process supported within *inclusive communities of participation*. These communities need to be understood as patterns of reflection, action and interaction.
- It *rejected team development as a linear process*. It is more complex than this. There is not one team development trajectory. Teams move back and forth, presenting and then discarding 'faces' according to the exigencies of the moment.
- It described the genesis and attributes of *three fundamental team 'faces'*:
  - face of the *emotionally literate team*;
  - face of the team that is *realistically optimistic*;
  - face of the team that *makes a difference*.
- *Changing faces* was accepted as normal and responsive to service demands and policy imperatives. Each change creates new team learning opportunities. These were regarded as *catalysts for further conversations of possibility*. Talking to learn is an essential part of developing a reflective team.
- It helped focus team members' attention and resources on matters significant to them and those with whom they work with and for whom they care. Teams *use their energies* (physical, mental, emotional, spiritual) in a *targeted and strategic manner*.

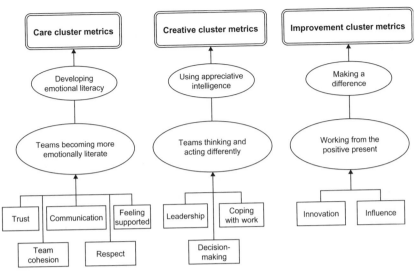

Figure 3.8 Evidence-based appreciative framework for supporting team-based r-learning (version 2) from a staff perspective. (After Ghaye 2005.)

Since then, and after working in more and different healthcare settings, things have matured. Although version 2 (Fig. 3.8) still contains many of the features of the original framework (see Fig. 1.4), some important improvements have been made. Figure 3.8 now holds some promise for helping us scale up r-learning through this particular action pathway named 'team'.

In summary, the improvements are as follows:

- R-learning brings more cohesion to the framework. Former reference to the practices of reflection are embedded within this.
- The 'attributes' of teams have been transformed into metrics.
- These metrics are now arranged into three clusters: care, creative and improvement clusters.
- Developing realistic optimism is now re-framed as 'using appreciative intelligence'.
- A newly validated care metric called 'respect' has been added. Reflection deleted.

Building a reflective organisation means that we need to:

- amplify the number of 'have moments' for staff;
- nurture the conditions for developing collective wisdom;
- actively draw upon open-space technology.

Progress along this action pathway symbolises progress towards building a reflective organisation.

Action pathway: network

In this section I explore the potential of scaling up r-learning through networks. As with other action pathways-to-scale, the positive core of this section is summarised in Table 0.3.

Networked organisations

NHS reforms in the UK, and the changing healthcare needs and expectations of the public, have given rise to a growing recognition of the need for new kinds of organisational structure and strategy. The networked organisation is one such response. The vocabulary of joint working, inter-professional learning, care pathways, inter-agency relations, joint ventures, organisational affiliation, public–private concordats, NHS collaboratives, integrated services, consortia, alliances and, of course, the dismantling of 'silos' clearly points to the fact that new organisational structures are providing opportunities to do different things and, I hope, to do things better.

> Networks in health and social care cover an eclectic variety of vertical and horizontal integration. These networks occur across a wide spectrum of agencies and individuals including purchasers, providers, professionals, and consumers. Moreover, networks in health and social care often have as their mission the wellbeing of users and patients . . . such networks are affected by societal values, egalitarianism and the 'public sector ethos', factors which may suggest the greater importance of solidarity and trust.

(Goodwin *et al.* 2004, p. 309).

In this section I focus essentially on scaling up r-learning through better intra-organisational networking, or, more precisely, by an 'appreciative sharing of knowledge' (Thatchenkery 2005) and skills through 'nets-that-work'.

In summary, the notion of a network implies nodes and links. The nodes can be individual people, teams or even whole organisations. Essentially, nodes are people. The links are the ways people interact with each other. A link may represent friendships, information flows (both face-to-face and electronic networks), the power to make decisions, various protocols and work agreement mechanisms, lines of reporting, and so on. Two-way links and reciprocity across the links are what make networks work.

There are many ways to classify types of network, for example by their:

- *Internal structure:* This includes the degree of centralisation (e.g. the presence of self-managing teams), the degree of density (e.g. the number of interactions between individuals and teams), the strength of links (e.g. formal or informal, professional or social), the extent of the structural equivalence between different parts of the network (e.g. the parts that have greater power to control budgets, make decisions, influence policy) and the extent to which the network is organised

into distinct clusters or cliques of high density linked by sparser ties
across its parts.

- *Content:* This refers to the nature of what is passed along the links that
  make up the network (e.g. information, capabilities, money, author-
  isation, emotional support). We can even map networks of resistance.
  More than one kind of thing can be passed along the same link.
- *Purpose:* This refers to the degree to which common tasks can be and
  actually are undertaken by members of the network (e.g. clinical, managerial, marketing). Wenger's (1998) notion of 'communities of practice' are social networks that facilitate ongoing knowledge sharing,
  discussion, mutual support and other social exchanges among affiliates
  who share an affinity to a particular profession or area of interest. The
  purpose of a network might be to provide or purchase services appropriate for patients, through integrated care pathways, to enable the
  sharing of scarce specialist human resources, or to share ideas and
  develop new technologies.
- *Ways of learning:* For example, we can think of networks of practitioners
  or teams that engage in r-learning. If a criterion for establishing a network is to encourage organisational innovation, then it is possible that
  learning is best promoted by network forms that exhibit a good deal of
  fluidity of membership and freedom for each organisation to terminate
  or replace particular nodes and links (Powell *et al.* 1996). All networks
  need to be reflective, embracing a continuous cycle of improvement.

Figure 3.9 is a schematic representation of the scaling up of r-learning
through networks. I have depicted this as a seven-part scaling-up process thus:

Schema 1
The individual reflective practitioner. Individuals may perceive themselves as 'lone workers' (e.g. practice nurse, osteopath, clinical bioethi-
cist). R-learning is undertaken as a private and solitary activity.

Schema 2
Loosely coupled professional acquaintances with a shared interest (e.g.
in practice nursing), but with little formal contact. Both schemas 1 and 2
are strongly regulated but weakly integrated. They are rarely involved in
networks. Again, r-learning is individualistic in kind. In schemas 1 and 2,
staff may be regarded as knowledgeable workers. They make the best
use of the knowledge and skills they possess. They are 'productive professionals' (Bryan & Joyce 2005, p. 1).

Schema 3
Hub-and-spoke interconnections and interdependencies. The hub can be
a clinical or team leader, while the spokes consist of individual clinicians
and other group members who are coupled more tightly or more loosely,
depending on their roles and responsibilities. Hub-and-spoke networks
can be scaled up. An example for the way services are organised for the
early intervention in psychosis could be like this: the reflective hub

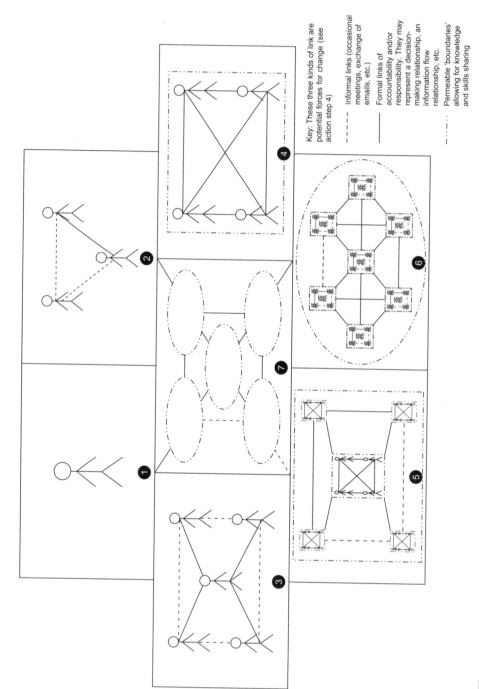

Key: These three kinds of link are potential forces for change (see action step 4)

- – – – Informal links (occasional meetings, exchange of emails, etc.)

———— Formal links of accountability and/or responsibility. They may represent a decision-making relationship, an information flow relationship, etc.

·–··–·· Permeable 'boundaries' allowing for knowledge and skills sharing

Figure 3.9 Schematic representation of the scaling up of r-learning through networks.

comprises a team manager, an employment adviser, a psychosocial therapies worker, an adolescent mental health practitioner and a clinical psychologist. The spokes could be made up from existing workers in the local community mental health trusts. Another example is that the reflective hub might be a public health intelligence (PHI) team that aims to serve a range of primary care trusts (PCTs) and a strategic health authority by using statistics intelligently to provide evidence of improvements in the health of the PCT population. The reflective hub would be the PHI nerve centre of information for the network, coordinating data on health inequalities, health needs assessment, equity audits, and so on. The (reflective) spokes involve PHI managers in PCTs; they are connected by such things as e-dialogue and monthly meetings. R-learning is a more collegial process.

Schema 4

The reflective team (Ghaye 2005), with a high level of team cohesion. Members make their learning and development visible to all staff. The focus is on team learning underpinned by forms of supported reflection and action. The emphasis is on learning and sharing for team development and service improvement. The interconnections and interdependencies enable reflective teams to be characterised as emotionally literate and appreciatively intelligent. They make an observable difference to practice and local policy. Scaled up, the 'team' may incorporate all those in a day case unit, in a head injury therapy unit, in a contraception and sexual health unit, in a neonatal intensive care unit, and so on. Reflective teams often have more distributed leadership, a great deal of social cohesion and explicit acknowledgement of shared values. R-learning is essentially among peers and undertaken publicly.

Schema 5

This scales up r-learning to the level of those within particular clinical or corporate directorates, for example within human resources (HR), where smaller units/teams such as those involved in HR policy and strategy, employee relations, occupational health, recruitment and retention, and so on, use r-learning.

Schema 6

This represents a scaling up of r-learning across directorates such as critical care, neurosciences, medicine, facilities, capital projects, finance, and information management and technology. In schemas 5 and 6, staff can reflect upon what might count as even better ways of working across poorly connected organisational silos. In schema 5, I suggest that, in certain circumstances, it might be useful to have a more 'offline' team (e.g. bottom left-hand corner) charged specifically with horizon-scanning and the discovery of new ideas and practices, and then reporting back more centrally.

Schema 7

Represents the way r-learning has been scaled up to an organisational level and shows reflective healthcare organisations linking with other health, social care and education providers within a particular strategic health authority.

Appreciative sharing of knowledge

In Thatchenkery (2005) and Thatchenkery & Choudhry (2007), we find the proposition that true knowledge sharing in organisations occurs less regularly than most of us think. So, if we wish knowledge of the intentions and achievements of r-learning to be scaled up through networks, so that it becomes an organisation-wide work habit, then a key question is 'What can be done to help create a kind of network that enables people to share their knowledge and experience of r-learning with others?'

Thatchenkery (2005) demonstrates how 'appreciation' is the missing link in facilitating this kind of knowledge sharing. He argues that by systematically and intentionally creating an appreciative culture within and between organisations, its leaders and practitioners are more likely to engage in the (appreciative) sharing of knowledge. He calls this process 'ASK': the appreciative sharing of knowledge combines *appreciative* inquiry, *social* constructionism and *knowledge* management. The goal of ASK is to identify the talents and competencies already at work in an organisation, to locate the good knowledge-sharing practices that already exist, and to enhance the values and behaviours that enable knowledge sharing to flourish.

Knowledge sharing is a relational activity

Knowledge sharing relies heavily on the nature, quality and quantity of direct and indirect interactions between people. To an extent, it also depends upon people's motivation, opportunity and ability to share knowledge. Arguably, networks are underpinned by values such as trust and egalitarianism. Knowledge is dynamically embedded in networks and processes, as well as in the human beings who constitute and use them. So if we are to use networks to scale up r-learning, then finding ways to make knowledge networks explicit is important. The reflective activity set out in Table 3.3 might be regarded as a first step to making such networks more explicit and known. When we know how they work and who is involved in them, we have a chance to use them to scale up knowledge about r-learning. Table 3.3 addresses a spectrum of interests from the individual to the collective, and from personal practice to organisational behaviour. Once entries in the 'Name' and 'Organisational location' columns have been made by a group of staff, they can set about creatively mapping the data as a pattern of nodes (people) and links. The latter need to be shown as labelled lines, which describe one (or more) of the ten knowledge-sharing interests, e.g. 'Trusting relationships'. The spatial arrangement of nodes needs to reflect the organisational location of each one. For example, those people working in the same directorate need to be shown as nodes in close proximity. I have found that the finished map of knowledge-sharing networks (the outcome) is not as important as the conversation staff have while generating it (the process).

When complete, and because of what it represents, the network map can be used as a catalyst for thinking and action about how it might be

Table 3.3 Ten reflective questions for mapping knowledge-sharing networks.

Knowledge-sharing about	Some reflective questions	Name of person(s)	Organisational location (e.g. directorate/ unit/dept/ward)
Organisational mission	With whom do you normally discuss the organisation's mission statement?		
Organisational values	With whom do you normally discuss what is important and valued in your organisation?		
What is happening	To whom do you normally go if you want to know what's going on at work?		
Professional qualities	Which people regularly appreciate your professional qualities?		
Trusting relationships	Who are the people with whom you have the most trusting relationships?		
Best practice	To whom do you normally go for expert advice?		
Personal performance	Whom do you normally seek out to get constructive feed-back on your work?		
Service user experiences	With whom do you normally discuss patient/client needs and wants?		
Innovation	With whom do you normally discuss better ways of doing things?		
Influence	To whom do you normally go if you want them to use their powers of persuasion and influence?		

best utilised to scale up r-learning. For example, it can be scanned for the presence (or absence) of 'enclave networks' (Goodwin *et al.* 2004) and decisions can then be made about the prudence of scaling up r-learning through them. Enclave networks are usually a close-knit group of staff with a high level of social cohesion. Additionally, members often have a common set of values. There is also a high level of internal equality between members and markedly less with outsiders.

> Such networks have great value, for example, in creating and developing 'bottom-up' legitimacy and trust between individuals, professionals and organisations to the sharing of information, ideas and strategies and to new ways of working.

(Goodwin *et al.* 2004, p. 77)

Summary

I have identified six possible and potentially useful action pathways (see Table 0.3). Earlier I talked about successful action being about choosing and following the most appropriate path. Successful action here means scaling up r-learning so that it becomes a collegial and useful organisation-wide work habit. Each action pathway enables us to make progress towards building a reflective healthcare organisation. What follows is a summary of the implications of following each pathway.

Action pathway: value

Building a reflective organisation means that a critical mass of staff need to subscribe to the shared value of engaging in collaborative forms of r-learning and doing this in a systematic, supported, rigorous and public manner.

Action pathway: conversation

Building a reflective organisation means that we need to:

- create the opportunity; and
- have the ability to use the power of the positive question to strengthen our collective capacity and capability to both imagine and build (even) better services for patients/clients.

Action pathway: user

Building a reflective organisation means that we need to sustain conversations of positive regard with service users through:

- trust
- engagement
- open and reflective listening
- feedback.

Progress along this action pathway requires us to ask the reflective questions 'What can I learn from service users' experience?' and 'How can this become an organisation-wide work habit?'

Action pathway: leadership

Building a reflective organisation means that we need to develop a critical mass of staff:

- with tipping-point leadership skills;
- who can exercise leadership with an appreciative eye;
- who can establish and sustain an appreciative disposition across the organisation;
- who work from the positive present.

Progress along this action pathway requires us to ask the reflective question 'How can we have more staff who can lead through appreciation?'

Action pathway: team

Building a reflective organisation means that we need to:

- amplify the number of 'have moments' for staff;
- nurture the conditions for developing collective wisdom;
- actively draw upon open space technology.

Action pathway: network

Building a reflective organisation means that we need to:

- understand how different kinds of network can be used to scale up r-learning;
- map and analyse the way knowledge-sharing networks develop and are sustained;
- view appreciative knowledge-sharing (ASK) networks as a key enabler to achieving scale.

References

Adler, M. & Fagley, N. (2005) Appreciation: individual differences in finding value and meaning as a unique predictor of subjective well-being. *Journal of Personality* 73(1), 79–114.

Anderson, H., Cooperrider, D., Gergen, K.J., et al. (2006) *The Appreciative Organization*. Taos Institute Publications, Chagrin Falls, OH.

Argyris, C. & Schön, D. (1974) *Theory in Practice: Increasing Professional Effectiveness*. Jossey-Bass, San Francisco, CA.

Argyris, C. & Schön, D. (1978) *Organizational Learning: A Theory of Action Perspective*. Addison Wesley, Reading, MA.

Argyris, C., Putnam, R. & McLain Smith, D. (1985) *Action Science: Concepts, Methods, and Skills for Research and Intervention*. Jossey-Bass, San Francisco, CA.

Belbin, M. (1982) *Management Teams: Why They Succeed or Fail*. Heinemann, London.

Bevan, H. (2006) On the push for productivity. *Health Service Journal*, 23 November, 26.

Blair, D. (2006) *Wittgenstein, Language and Information: 'Back to the Rough Ground!'* Springer-Verlag, New York.

Branthwaite, M. (2005) Taking the final step: changing the law on euthanasia and physician assisted suicide. *British Medical Journal* **331**, 681–3.

Bryan, L. & Joyce, C. (2005) The 21st century organisation. *McKinsey Quarterly* **3**, 24–33.

Carlisle, D. (2006) Outside edge: leadership. *Health Service Journal*, 15 June, 34.

Carr, D. (1992) Practical enquiry, values and the problem of educational theory. *Oxford Review of Education* **18**(3), 241–51.

Chaffee, P. (2005) *Claiming the Light: Appreciative Inquiry & Corporate Transformation.* Alban Books, Herndon, VA.

Collins, J. (2001) *Good to Great: Why Some Companies Make the Leap . . . and Others Don't.* HarperBusiness, New York.

Collins, J. (2006) *Good to Great and the Social Sectors.* Random House Business Books, London.

Commission for Health Improvement (2003). *A Report on the NHS: Getting Better?* Commission for Health Improvement, London.

Cooperrider, D. (2001) Appreciative inquiry: releasing the power of the positive question. Working paper. Case Western Reserve University, Cleveland, OH. Available at http://appreciativeinquiry.case.edu/uploads/working_paper_AI_and_power_positive_question.pdf

Cooperrider, D. & Srivastva, S. (1987) Appreciative inquiry in organizational life. In *Research in Organizational Change and Development*, Vol. 1 (eds W.A. Pasmore & R.W. Woodman). JAI Press, Greenwich, CT.

Cooperrider, D. & Whitney, D. (1999) *Appreciative Inquiry: Collaborating for Change.* Berrett-Koehler, San Francisco, CA.

Cooperrider, D. & Whitney, D. (2005) *Appreciative Inquiry: A Positive Revolution in Change.* Berrett-Koehler, San Francisco, CA.

Cooperrider, D., Whitney, D. & Stavros, J.M. (2003) *Appreciative Inquiry Handbook.* Lakeshore Publishers, Bedford Heights, OH.

Cooperrider, D., Sorensen, P.F. & Yaeger, T. (eds) (2005) *Appreciative Inquiry: An Emerging Direction for Organization Development.* Stipes Publishing, Champaign, IL.

Coulter, A. & Ellins, J. (2006) *Patient-Focused Interventions: A Review of the Evidence.* Health Foundation and the Picker Institute Europe, London. Available at: www.pickereurope.org/Filestore/Downloads/QEI-Review-intro.pdf

Davies, H. (2002) Understanding organizational culture in reforming the National Health Service. *Journal of the Royal Society of Medicine* **95**(3), 140–42.

Department of Health (2001) *Working Together – Learning Together: A Framework for Lifelong Learning in the NHS.* Department of Health, London.

Department of Health (2002a) *Liberating the Talents: Helping Primary Care Trusts and Nurses to Deliver the NHS Plan.* Department of Health, London.

Department of Health (2002b) *Shifting the Balance of Power: The Next Steps.* Department of Health, London.

Department of Health (2002c) *Improving Working Lives for the Allied Health Professions and Healthcare Scientists.* Department of Health, London.

Department of Health (2003) *Delivering the Best: Midwives Contribution to the NHS Plan.* Department of Health, London. Available at www.publications.doh.gov.uk/cno/midwives.pdf

Department of Health (2004) *National Service Framework for Children, Young People and Maternity Services: Executive Summary.* Department of Health, London. Available at: www.dh.gov.uk/PublicationsAndStatistics/Publications/PublicationsPolicy AndGuidance/PublicationsPolicyAndGuidanceArticle/fs/en?CONTENT_ID=4089100&chk=Egpznc

Fisman, R. & Khanna, T. (1999) Is trust a historical residue? Information flows and trust levels. *Journal of Economic Behaviour and Organisation* **38**(1), 79–92.

Folkman, J.R. (2006) *The Power of Feedback: 35 Principles for Turning Feedback from Others into Personal and Professional Change*. John Wiley & Sons, Princeton, NJ.

Gadsby, A. (2006) If service users felt listened to they'd be happier to compromise. *Nursing Times* **47**, 10.

Gardner, H. (1993) *Frames of Mind: The Theory of Multiple Intelligences*. Basic Books, New York.

Gergen, K. (1994) *Realities and Relationships*. Harvard University Press, Cambridge, MA.

Gerteis, M., Edgman-Levitan, S., Daley, J. & Delbanco, T.L. (eds) (1993) *Through the Patient's Eyes*. Jossey-Bass, San Francisco, CA.

Ghaye, T. (2005) *Developing the Reflective Healthcare Team*. Blackwell Publishing, Oxford.

Ghaye, T. & Lillyman, S. (eds) (2000) *Caring Moments: The Discourse of Reflective Practice*. Quay Books, Salisbury.

Ghaye, T. & Lillyman, S. (2001) *Learning Journals and Critical Incidents: Reflective Practice for Health Care Professionals*. Quay Books, Salisbury.

Gladwell, M. (2005) *The Tipping Point: How Little Things Can Make A Big Difference*. Abacus, London.

Goldhammer, R. (1966) A Critical Analysis Of Supervision Of Instruction in the Harvard–Lexington Summer Programme. PhD thesis, Harvard University, Cambridge, MA.

Goodwin, N., 6, P., Peck, E., *et al.* (2004) Managing across diverse networks of care: lessons from other sectors. Report to the National Co-ordinating Centre for NHS Service Delivery and Organisation R & D (NCCSDO). Available at www.sdo.lshtm.ac.uk/files/adhoc/39-policy-report.pdf

Gould, M. (2003) NHS star rating system is misleading, statisticians say. *British Medical Journal* **327**, 1008.

Heifetz, R. & Linsky, M. (2002) *Leadership on the Line: Staying Alive through the Dangers of Leading*. Harvard Business School Press, Boston, MA.

Higgs, J. & Titchen, A. (2001) *Professional Practice in Health, Education and the Creative Arts*. Blackwell Science, Oxford.

Hofstede, G. (1994) *Cultures and Organisations: Software of the Mind*. HarperCollins, London.

Hunt, C. & Sampson, F. (1998) *The Self on the Page*. Jessica Kingsley Publishers, London.

Kahane, A. (2004) *Solving Tough Problems*. Berrett-Koehler, San Francisco, CA.

Kember, D., Jones, A., Loke, A.Y., *et al.* (2001) *Reflective Teaching and Learning in the Health Professions*. Blackwell Science, Oxford.

Kidder, R.M. (2005) *Moral Courage*. W. Morrow, New York.

Kim, C. & Mauborgne, R. (2003) Tipping point leadership. *Harvard Business Review*, April, 60–69.

Kur, E. (1996) The faces model of high performing team development. *Management Development Review* **9**(6), 25–35.

Lewis, R., Hunt, P. & Carson, D. (2006) Social enterprise and community-based care. Working paper. Kings Fund, London.

Maternity Care Working Party (2006) *Modernising Maternity Care: A Commissioning Toolkit for Primary Care Trusts in England*. Maternity Care Working Party, London. Available at: www.nct.org.uk/files/downloads/mmctoolkit06.pdf

Melander-Wikman, A., Jansson, M. & Ghaye, T. (2006) Reflections on an appreciative approach to empowering elderly people in home healthcare. *Reflective Practice* **7**(4), 423–44.

Meleis, A.F. (1996). Culturally competent scholarship: substance and rigor. *Advances in Nursing Science* **19**(2), 1–16.

Miller, D. (1990) *The Icarus Paradox*. HarperCollins, New York.

Mills, C. (2005). *NHS Reform: Consumerism or Citizenship?* Mutuo, London.

Morgan, G. (2006) *Images of Organization*. Sage, Thousand Oaks, CA.

NHS Modernisation Agency (2004) *Survey of Models of Maternity Care: Towards Sustainable WTD Compliant Staffing and Clinical Network Solutions.* NHS Modernisation Agency, London. Available at: www.rcog.org.uk/resources/Public/pdf/survey_of_models_maternity_care.pdf

Novak, J. (1998) *Learning, Creating and Using Knowledge.* Lawrence Erlbaum, London.

Nursing and Midwifery Council (2002) *Supporting Nurses and Midwives through Lifelong Learning.* Nursing and Midwifery Council, London.

O'Dowd, A. (2006) A motivational scheme at a London hospital encourages nurses to be helpful and friendly to patients. *Nursing Times* **102**(45), 9.

Owen, H. (1997) *Open Space Technology.* Berrett-Koehler, San Francisco, CA.

Parkinson, F. (1997) *Critical Incident Debriefing: Understanding and Dealing with Trauma.* Souvenir Press, London.

Plsek, P.E. & Wilson, T. (2001) Complexity science: complexity, leadership, and management in healthcare organisations. *British Medical Journal* **323**, 746–9.

Polanyi, M. (1958) *Personal Knowledge.* Oxford University Press, Oxford.

Powell, W., Koput, K. & Smith-Doerr, L. (1996) Inter-organisational collaboration and the locus of innovation: networks of learning in biotechnology. *Administrative Science Quarterly* **41**, 116–45.

Putnam, R.D., Leonardi, R. & Nanetti, R. (1993) *Making Democracy Work: Civic Traditions in Modern Italy.* Princeton University Press, Princeton, NJ.

Reina, D. & Reina, M. (2006) *Trust and Betrayal in the Workplace: Building Effective Relationships in Your Organisation.* Berrett-Koehler, San Francisco, CA.

Robertson Cooper Ltd (2006) *Teamable: Making your Teamwork.* Available at: www.robertsoncooper.com/products/Teamable.aspx

Rothstein, B. (2000), Trust, social dilemmas and collective memories. *Journal of Theoretical Politics* **12**(4), 477–501.

Schiller, M., Mah Holland, B. & Riley, D. (eds) (2001) *Appreciative Leaders: In the Eye of the Beholder.* Taos Institute Publications, Chagrin Falls, OH.

Sensky, T. (2002) Withdrawal of life sustaining treatment. *British Medical Journal* **325**, 175–6.

Srivastva, S., Cooperrider, D. & Case Western Reserve University (eds) (1990) *Appreciative Leadership and Management.* Jossey-Bass, San Francisco, CA.

Stavros, J. & Torres, C. (2005) *Dynamic Relationships: Unleashing the Power of Appreciative Inquiry in Daily Living.* Taos Institute Publications, Chagrin Falls, OH.

Surowiecki, J. (2004) *The Wisdom of Crowds.* Doubleday, New York.

Thatchenkery, T. (2005) *Appreciative Sharing of Knowledge: Leveraging Knowledge Management for Strategic Change.* Taos Institute Publications, Chagrin Falls, OH.

Thatchenkery, T. & Choudhry, D. (2007) *Appreciative Inquiry and Knowledge Management: A Social Constructionist Perspective.* Edward Elgar Publishing, Cheltenham.

Thatchenkery, T. & Metzker, C. (2006) *Appreciative Intelligence: Seeing the Mighty Oak in the Acorn.* Berrett-Koehler, San Francisco, CA.

Tuckman, B.W. (1965) Development sequence in small groups. *Psychological Bulletin* **63**, 384–99.

Van de Ven, A.H., Polley, D., Garud, R. & Venkataraman. S. (1999) *The Innovation Journey.* Oxford University Press, New York and Oxford.

van Manen, M. (1997) *Researching Lived Experience: Human Science for an Action Sensitive Pedagogy.* SUNY Press, New York.

Wenger, E. (1998) *Communities of Practice: Learning, Meaning and Identity.* Cambridge University Press, Cambridge.

Wheatley, M.J. (2002) *Turning to One Another: Simple Conversations to Restore Hope to the Future.* Berrett-Koehler, San Francisco, CA.

Whitehead, J. (1993) *The Growth Of Educational Knowledge: Creating Your Own Living Educational Theories.* Hyde Publications, Bournemouth.

Whitehead, J. (2000) How do I improve my practice? Creating and legitimating an epistemology of practice. *Reflective Practice* **1**(1), 91–104.

Whitehead, J., with Johns, C. (2000) A response to Whitehead, and a reply. *Reflective Practice* **1**(1), 105–12.

Whitney, D. & Trosten-Bloom, A. (2002) *The Power of Appreciative Inquiry.* Berrett-Koehler, San Francisco, CA.

Whitney, D., Cooperrider, D., Trosten-Bloom, A. & Kaplan, B. (2002) *The Encyclopedia of Positive Questions.* Lakeshore Communications, Euclid, OH.

Whitney, D., Trosten-Bloom, A., Cherney, J. & Fry, R. (2005) *Appreciative Team Building.* iUniverse, New York.

Chapter 4

Action step 4: a force for change

Up to this point, I have tried to set out clearly a vision for a healthcare organisation with reflective characteristics. Additionally, I have re-framed reflective practice as r-learning and described its four principle intentions. In the previous chapter, I tried to take you safely over some of the 'rough ground' to be found along six action pathways-to-scale. In doing so, I have suggested that successful journeying might enable you to scale up r-learning so that it becomes a collegial and useful, organisation-wide work habit. In this final action step, I set out a practical force for change that helps us to build a reflective healthcare organisation. In its totality, I call this RAISE. It is grounded in practice and developed from work undertaken from both inside and beyond healthcare. It is, therefore, eclectic in origin and positive in intent.

RAISE

In the introduction to this book, I mentioned briefly that RAISE is a force for change with two meanings. First, it is a word in its own right with a clear action orientation. It is meant to convey a sense of raising people's courage and spirits in order to adopt a more persistent, strengths-based approach to service improvement and organisational development, reflecting on and learning from strengths, rather than failings and failures. Second, RAISE is an acronym. Its components describe five forces that need to operate to give us the much needed momentum to progress along one or more action pathways-to-scale. In summary, the five forces that comprise RAISE are as follows:

R = reflecting
Systematically, rigorously, supportively and publicly learning from reflecting on our practice. The driving force begins with developing positive appreciations. This takes us in the direction of positive action.
A = appreciating
This is a force in two parts: appreciating how people and organisational cultures serve to liberate or constrain us, and appreciating how articulating individual, team and organisational 'best practices' provides a constructive force for creating a positive vision of the future.
I = interacting
This essentially refers to how we can shift away from interacting using reloading and downloading habits (see p. 16) to interactions that are fuelled by reflective, generative and transformational conversations

(see pp. 14–15) – in a nutshell, more hopeful conversations. Learned optimism and the power of the positive question are important elements. But, as I will explain later, this force is also about using 'non-negative thinking' (Seligman 2006).

S = strategising

Scaling up r-learning requires a strategy. Whereas 'strategy' refers to content (e.g. 'the strategy'), 'strategising' refers to the process of strategy formation (Jarzabkowski 2005). The word includes the practices available for shaping it, together with an understanding of the consequences of that shaping. Inevitably, strategising is linked to the notion of power as understood by Foucault (1977). Power (or the lack of it) is a potent force. It influences strategic action.

E = energising

Making progress in building a reflective healthcare organisation requires energy. Energy management and renewal are, therefore, important strategies in making this a healthy pursuit (Redwood *et al.* 1999). The need for recovery is not a sign of weakness but an integral part of staying focused and making progress along the action pathways of our choice. Great conversations can be energising. Working towards an ambitious goal can also be energising. Reflecting on our energy levels (over- and underuse) is essential because energy (i.e. not just time) is essential in building the reflective organisation. Different kinds of energy provide a different force for change.

Illustrating RAISE in practice

The results of a comprehensive process of 'discovery' (Cooperrider & Whitney 2005) undertaken by the Institute of Reflective Practice in 2005 into working life in maternity services in a part of the UK are shown in Fig. 4.1. Data for this were gathered via a specially designed workplace culture and team wellness questionnaire called STEPs (Institute of Reflective Practice UK 2007). A total of 702 questionnaires were returned. At that time, the results were presented back to staff at 31 separate meetings, in 10 different NHS trusts, over a 2-month period. Figure 4.1 shows that at that time, the findings were couched as 'high-impact changes'. Changing existing patterns of behaviours to improve multidisciplinary team working was the top priority in each of the ten participating hospitals. In our meetings with staff, most conversations were about the link between multidisciplinary team work and:

- client safety
- roles and responsibilities
- communication
- leadership
- shared learning opportunities
- working relationships.

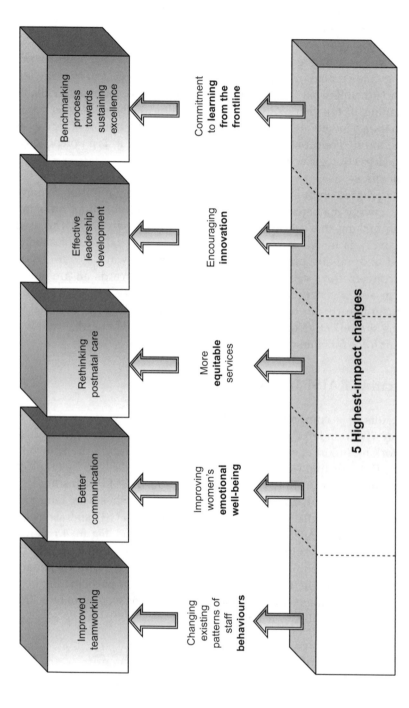

Figure 4.1 Appreciating the 'problems' in maternity services and linking this with action.

The data and the conversations gave us all much to reflect upon. It had certainly deepened our appreciation of the 'problems' facing maternity services in that part of the UK. But with some re-framing, the challenge became clear: improving services for woman was essentially about improving patterns of staff behaviour. Put another way, it was about relationships. This was not the message everyone wanted to hear. There were other, more dominant and more pervasive languages being used at that time. For example, the languages of:

- the cost of increasing clinical activity;
- the increasing clinical dependency of women;
- the physical capacity of services;
- cappings and bookings;
- midwifery agency usage;
- the age profile of midwives.

Although big changes were needed, big change began with trying to get r-learning to 'stick' to individuals. Kahane (2004) eloquently puts it this way:

> There is a story about a man who wanted to change the world. He tried as hard as he could, but really did not accomplish anything. So he thought that instead he should just try to change his country, but he had no success with that either. Then he tried to change his city and then his neighbourhood, still unsuccessfully. Then he thought that he could at least change his family, but failed again. So he decided to change himself. Then a surprising thing happened. As he changed himself, his family changed too. And as his family changed, his neighbourhood changed. As his neighbourhood changed, his city changed. As his city changed, his country changed, and as his country changed, the world changed.

(Kahane 2004, p. 131)

During 2006, and armed with these appreciations, Institute staff began a series of supportive workshops inside the different units using the RAISE process. What follows are some illustrations of the way RAISE became a positive force for change. Some activities and outcomes are presented. Reading with an appreciative eye should enable you to spot how:

- the four intentions of r-learning were brought to life in this context;
- staff journeyed along different action pathways;
- problems and deficit-based conversations were re-framed;
- staff were able to establish the 'positive core' for their services;
- a more positive future could unfold from the present;
- RAISE enabled r-learning to 'spread' and 'stick' with more and more staff and in different organisations, across the year.

R = *reflecting*

The basic r-learning intentions depicted in Fig. 0.2 provided us with our starting point. Knowing what we knew then, we began by asking

Table 4.1 The four intentions of r-learning, potential barriers and barrier-busting appreciative questions.

Basic r-learning intention	Potential barrier to realising the intention	Barrier-busting appreciative question
1 Developing appreciation	Failure to 'feel'	Think of an occasion when you felt valued by those with whom you work. What do you need to do to feel this way again?
2 Re-framing experience	Failure to 'see'	Think of a moment when you realised 'There are other ways to do or understand this.' What do you need to do to experience this again?
3 Building collective wisdom	Failure to 'share'	Think of a time, at work, when you could meet, talk and learn with your colleagues. What do you need to do to create this time again?
4 Acknowledging achievement	Failure to 'move'	Think of the last time you were supported in your efforts to move your knowledge and skills forward. What do you need to do to achieve this kind of support again?

ourselves the question 'What kinds of things are likely to get in the way of realising each of the intentions of r-learning?' These are shown in the central column in Table 4.1. We then asked ourselves 'How could we re-frame these problems and transform them into 'barrier-busting questions' that we could invite staff to engage with?' These are shown in Table 4.1.

Of course, re-framing problems, even with the best barrier-busting questions at hand, is no easy task. We need not only the ability to do this but also the commitment. Tough problems, according to Kahane (2004), are so because they are complex in three ways. They are:

- *Dynamically complex:* This means that the causes of the problem, and its effects on people, processes and things, are far apart in space and time.

- *Generatively complex:* This means that the problems unfold in an unfamiliar and unpredictable manner. Their origin surprises us. Their effects catch us out. Solutions to problems with this kind of complexity cannot be calculated in advance. Solutions cannot be worked out based on what may have happened in the past, but have to be worked out as the situation unfolds.
- *Socially complex:* This means that the people involved with this problem see things very differently. As problems get unpicked, either they grow in size or views about their causes and effects become polarised. In these situations, conversations get stuck.

To solve a complex problem, we have to immerse ourselves in and open up to its full complexity. Dynamic complexity requires us to not just talk with the experts close to us, but also with people on the periphery. Generative complexity requires that we talk not only about options that worked in the past, but also about ones that are emerging now. And social complexity requires us to talk not just with people who see things the same way we do, but especially with those who see things differently, even those we don't like. We must stretch way beyond our comfort zone.

(Kahane 2004, p. 75)

A = appreciation

With staff across the different organisations, we invited them to undertake some appreciative pairs work (see p. 192). We introduced this thus: We opened with a negative statement, in the hope that it would, after explanation, be viewed as a positive statement. The negative was what we did *not* want them to do – that is, to go around the circle, introducing themselves to one another in turn. What we *did* want them to do was to introduce someone else in the circle to the group. They were free to choose who, but they had to make sure that everyone was introduced. This was their collective responsibility. Sometimes they had to be creative in being responsible in this way if there were new or unfamiliar staff in the circle. We gave them some thinking time. Each introduction had to follow a similar pattern. It was the person's name followed by an appreciative statement about a particular personal or professional quality, gift or talent the 'other' had. Table 4.2 shows what one multidisciplinary group thought of each other. After the introductions have been made, we always ask two questions: 'What did that feel like for you?' and 'What did you think when you heard what another person thinks of you?' These questions not only set the tone for forthcoming interactions but also help everyone appreciate a range of issues about, for example, self-presentation, self-awareness, the accuracy of self-assessment, self-confidence and relationship management.

The 'bettering' activity

Another way we use the force of appreciations is through a reflective group task that we call 'bettering'. More precisely, it is triggered by the

Table 4.2   Developing appreciations of one another.

Name	What we appreciate about our colleague
Tracey	Has a wonderful way of sorting out problems. She gives me ideas. Very good with mothers – they feel appreciated.
Pauline	She is always patient and understanding. She keeps people motivated and is an excellent role model.
Amy	She is always cheerful, conscientious and a good decision-maker. She really understands women.
Jez	She is very flexible and grabs the job at hand immediately. She is my mentor.
Bev	She has a gentle and calming approach.
Holly	She brings a warm presence around the place. She is a pleasure to be around. She has a fantastic smile that lifts all the staff on the ward.
Elsie	Very good at passing on information. She is great with all the mums.
Mary	She has made a lot of difference. She keeps the paediatricians in order! She loves babies and supports mothers.
Ginger	She always seems to be able to solve my problems and see things differently.
Sandra	She is so full of energy. She is extremely helpful and sorts out all the problems.

statement 'What I'd like to know more about you, so that I can work even better with you', hence the use of the term 'bettering'. Staff are invited to get into small groups. Each person is then given a number of pieces of paper that match the number of people in the group. Time is given for each member to write a number of personal responses to the statement, one for each member sitting in their circle or around their table. Papers are then folded and placed in front of the appropriate person, so each member of the group ends up with a small pile of folded papers that they are then asked to read. They do this quietly and privately. They are asked to reflect on what they are thinking and feeling while doing this, and to select one written response that is either:

- significant to them in some way; and/or
- achievable.

   Without any coercion, staff are then invited to read out one (or more) of their chosen statements to others in their group. No responses or comments are allowed at this time, as this part of the activity calls for open

Box 4.1   Some evidence from the 'bettering' activity

'What I'd like to know more about you so that I can work even better with you':

Paula received:
- What motivates you and how do you see your role?
- How do you stay so calm?
- How are you so patient?
- Like to know your sense of humour and how you cope with a very busy day.

Sandy received:
- What makes you smile?
- How do you cope with being a deputy manager?
- How do you manage to stay so positive about the staff with the increasing numbers of patient complaints?
- How do I know your thanks is real?

Jasna received:
- What makes you happy to be so open with people?
- What makes you irritable?
- What do you want for your future?
- How do you stay so relaxed?

Trish received:
- How would you feel if you came into the wards more often?
- What makes you happy?
- What do you do in your office all day?
- How do you feel when staff come to see you with their problems?

Jill received:
- Why don't you seem to realise how important your input is seen to be?
- What made you take such a big career change?
- What motivates you?
- Have you got your heart in your job?

and reflective listening. Box 4.1 shows some of the outcomes to this activity. Staff were in groups of five.

Through whole-group discussion, we try to make some sense of the experience to date. We then try to go on to co-construct some 'themes' that serve to summarise what has been written down, for example 'What I think', 'How I feel', 'How my behaviours impact on others', and so on. At this point, we pick one theme, for example 'The impact of your behaviours on others'. We then invite staff: 'Try to recall a positive experience, in the recent past, related to the impact of your behaviours on others'. On a separate piece of paper they write down:

- what it was;
- what made it a positive experience;
- what they need to do more of.

Box 4.2 shows responses from three staff.

Box 4.2 Appreciating the root causes of success and action to amplify this

What was it?

- Situation that was deteriorating (low staff morale, and moaning). Member of staff identified the unpleasant working environment and called staff together to tackle problems and moods. After confrontation and communication, the working environment became positive and pleasant.
- Being nominated for staff awards.
- Helping a woman frightened at prospect of giving birth.

What made it positive?

- Early identification of problems. Dealt with earlier, which prevented festering negativity. Stopped people feeling negative for rest of shift. Made staff think about their mood and impact on each other. Facilitated an environment for the staff to talk to each other.
- Wasn't expecting it – made me feel like I wanted to do more. Opposite of impression that others thought of you.
- Alleviated her fears.

What do you need to do more of?

- Talk to each other. Try to have a positive way of thinking about each. Team playing. Be more open with each other and not feel intimidated by doing so.
- Consider impact of comments. Give ongoing positive feedback. Go directly to source.
- Be accurate/appropriate with information:
  - listen;
  - educate;
  - agree plan of care;
  - communicate – open channel;
  - follow up and feed back.

These activities give staff experience of engaging in r-learning. They also opened the way for a productive conversation, underpinned by the theory of personal control about:

- their ability to think positively;
- their power of 'non-negative thinking' when they feel things are going less well than they had hoped;
- the quality of their interpersonal relationships.

Perspectives from positive psychology

Seligman (2006) reminds us how important learned helplessness and explanatory style are to understanding working life (e.g. healthcare practice) as successes or failures of personal control:

> Learned helplessness is the giving up reaction, the quitting response that follows from the belief that whatever you do doesn't matter. Explanatory style is the manner in which you habitually explain to yourself why events happen . . . An optimistic explanatory style stops helplessness, whereas a pessimistic explanatory style spreads helplessness. Your way of explaining events to yourself determines how helpless you can become, or how energized . . .

(Seligman 2006, pp. 15–16)

In a very cogent way, Seligman (2006) argues that there is one particularly self-defeating way to think, namely making personal, permanent and pervasive explanations for bad events. Pessimists believe that bad events will last a long time, will undermine everything they do and are their own fault. RAISE is a force for optimism. Through collegial forms of reflection, failures to meet targets or clinical outcomes being less good than hoped for can be put into perspective. Just like we can learn to be helpless, so too can we learn to be optimistic.

I = interacting and S = strategising

These are both powerful forces for change. I illustrate them with reference to staff members, in multiple hospital sites, who were engaging in r-learning. R-learning was being scaled up largely by progress along three action pathways simultaneously. They were the 'Values', 'Conversation' and 'User' pathways. Staff in each maternity unit were invited to think about a woman whom they felt had a positive and successful postnatal experience in their unit. They were asked to discuss this woman's experience within a group. They were then asked to write down their responses with regard to five postnatal care metrics. These metrics were aspects of care that women regarded as being particularly important to them. The results from one group of staff are shown in Table 4.3. The principal forces at work here were interacting and strategising

Table 4.3 Making successful progress along the values, conversation and user action pathways.

Reflective invitation	Support from staff	Postnatal care metrics			
		Quality time	Coping with vulnerability	Involvement	Privacy and dignity
1 'We know this was a particularly positive experience for this woman because . . .'	We received feedback from the mother both while she was in hospital and once at home	Of the gratitude she expressed on the level of care given to her baby while in FCU. Positive feedback from extended family	She returned to the ward with a card and gift to say thank you, as baby was still breastfeeding, gaining weight and thriving 3 months later	She was a first-time mum who had no idea of 'what to do with herself and her baby'	Verbal feedback from her was positive
2 'We think the reasons for the woman's experience being so positive are . . .'	Support and help from all members of staff. Pleasant approach from staff. Mother given practical help and advice	The staff's awareness of the woman's condition and how precious her baby was in the family network. Effective communication with the family	Because she felt supported, listened to and helped to establish breastfeeding	Staff involvement of mother and partner in the care, e.g. breast-feeding, nappy changing, bath demonstration. Encouraging mother to request	Because care was tailored to her individual needs, e.g. confidential, sensitive information about her remained private and she was treated in a

		and a good personal relationship with the family		pain relief and help when needed. Advice on hygiene, diet and postnatal exercises	non-judgemental way
3 'Learning from this woman's experience means we need to do more . . .'	Listening to the woman's needs. Continuing to provide staff who are able to support and assist. Staff to encourage women's self-confidence	To continue to be aware that every woman has individual needs. To maintain good communication skills with the family. This is paramount	Listening, supporting and assisting women in the early point of postnatal care to achieve successful breast-feeding and parenting skills	Supervision of parental skills and offer help with care when necessary	Identifying individual needs/ sensitive issues. Ensuring we always treat women in a non-judgemental way
4 'This means we need to . . .'	Communicate the plan of care with each mother and other members of multidisciplinary team	Maintain and improve communica-tion skills with each other and families/ better teamwork. Increase staff levels and support workers to allow more time with clients	Prioritise and focus more on the women whose needs are greater	Reflect on our practice and success and maintain it	Listen to women in order to understand what their individual needs are

forces. One outcome was the eventual emergence of a positive core. It read:

> Our maternity unit is an environment where we provide optimum care, on an individual basis, by listening to women in a non-judgemental way and identifying their needs in a culture of mutual respect.

Under this positive core was the statement:

So this means we need to:

- reflect on our practice and success, as a multidisciplinary team;
- work as a team to respond positively to women's individual needs.

E = energising

As explained earlier, strategising refers to the process of strategy formation and includes the practices available for shaping it. Strategising requires energy. In Box 4.3 we find some of the documented outcomes of

---

Box 4.3   Some documented outcomes of the process of strategising

- Know our purpose/vision/aim. Share positive experience. Recognise and reward hard work. Promote individual support (flexible working hours). Have approachable/supportive leadership. Define our goal.
- Keep improving communication. Respect each other and what we do, to keep encouraging each other. How do we put it into practice?
- Think positive! Reflect on what's being discussed. Move forward in order to achieve what we've learnt today. Spread the words!
- Feed back all service users' comments to staff. Involve staff in decision-making. Have time available for support for staff. Treat colleagues with respect.
- Communicate more effectively. Be there for each other. Listen and acknowledge others' actions. Give praise and say thank you. Develop more multidisciplinary team cohesion.
- Spend more quality time together where possible in a less stressful, less formal environment in order to appreciate each other better and learn from each other and form a closer and more respectful bond.
- Nurture what is good with respect. Build on what makes a good team. Listen to each other in a positive way. Give each other support.
- Be approachable and well informed of all the changes and keep up to date with present information. More support (visible) from management.

the strategising undertaken by the staff group who produced Table 4.3. Through discussion with them, four different kinds of energy were working, differentially, to provide the force for achieving such outcomes. They were:

- *Emotional energy:* Generated by the positive feelings of mutual appreciation experienced by staff as they engaged in the activity.
- *Physical energy:* The amount of physical energy they could devote to interacting and strategising, and especially given that many staff that day were juggling numerous commitments.
- *Mental energy:* The way staff found the mental energy to stay focused, for long enough, and without distraction from other duties, to feel they were actually achieving something and moving forward. This is the fourth intention of r-learning (see Fig. 0.2).
- *Spiritual energy:* Energy derived through interacting with others in a safe and supportive context and from achieving deeper appreciations of the alignment of their espoused values and their values-in-action.

The scaling up of r-learning, so that it becomes a collegial and useful, organisation-wide work habit, requires the full engagement of everyone. As Loehr & Schwartz (2005) explain, it is energy, not time, that is the fundamental currency of achieving this kind of goal

> To be fully engaged, we must be physically energized, emotionally connected, mentally focused and spiritually aligned with a purpose beyond our immediate self-interest.

(Loehr & Schwartz 2005, p. 5)

Loehr & Schwartz (2005) set out four key management principles that they believe are at the heart of any change process. They are:

- Full engagement requires drawing on four separate but related sources of energy: physical, emotional, mental and spiritual.
- Because energy capacity diminishes both with overuse and with underuse, we must balance energy expenditure with intermittent energy renewal.
- To build capacity, we must push beyond our normal limits, training in the same systematic way that elite athletes do.
- Positive energy rituals (highly specific routines for managing energy) are the key to full engagement and sustained high performance.

RAISE describes five forces that need to operate in order to give us the much needed momentum to progress along one or more action pathways-to-scale. But what is this experience like? What do staff learn as they journey over their 'rough ground'? In Box 4.4 I include eight responses from one group of staff who were committed to building a reflective healthcare organisation through r-learning. It was early days for them. Here were their answers to the question 'What is the most important thing you've learned today?'

Box 4.4   What is the most important thing you've learned today?

- Positive thinking. Build on what we are doing well. Open-minded. Supportive to one another.
- Be appreciative of, and supportive to, each other to have a more effective team.
- I have learnt that we should value each member of staff who contributes to a safe, happy, supportive work environment.
- To focus on the positive for it to increase.
- To be supportive, appreciative and respectful in our working environment in order to achieve effective teamwork. Also not forgetting and communicating effectively.
- The importance of teamwork, and why colleagues should be respected, appreciated and acknowledged.
- To appreciate my colleagues more and see their strengths and positive sides and communicate better with them.
- The team has to use the head (knowledge), hand (doing) and heart (feeling) in harmony (balance) for it to be successful.

References

Cooperrider, D. & Whitney, D. (2005) *Appreciative Inquiry: A Positive Revolution in Change*. Berrett-Koehler, San Francisco, CA.

Foucault, M. (1977) *Discipline and Punish*. Tavistock, London.

Institute of Reflective Practice-UK (2007) *STEPs*. IRP-UK Publications, Gloucester.

Jarzabkowski, P. (2005) *Strategy as Practice: An Activity-Based Approach*. Sage Publications, London.

Kahane, A. (2004) *Solving Tough Problems*. Berrett-Koehler, San Francisco, CA.

Loehr, J. & Schwartz, T. (2005) *The Power of Full Engagement*. The Free Press, New York.

Redwood, S., Goldwasser, C., Street, S. & PricewaterhouseCoopers LLP (1999) *Action Management*. John Wiley & Sons, New York.

Seligman, M. (2006) *Learned Optimism: How to Change Your Mind and Your life*. Vintage Books, New York.

Summary

This book has been about building the reflective healthcare organisation by acting with appreciative intent.

Useful metaphors

Two metaphors have been used to help make sense of this complex process. They are:

- Van de Ven's metaphor of a 'journey';
- Wittgenstein's metaphor of 'rough ground'.

The central question

How can we scale up r-learning so that it becomes a collegial and useful, organisation-wide, sustainable work habit?

R-learning

Reflective practice has been re-framed as reflective learning (r-learning). The four intentions of r-learning are:

- developing appreciations of one's own and others' feelings, thoughts and quality of action;
- re-framing experience so that we can better understand our conviction-laden practices and create new and improved realities;
- building collective wisdom through conversations of positive regard;
- achieving and moving forward, appreciating how a better future unfolds from the positive present.

Action pathways-to-scale

Six action pathways-to-scale have been presented. Each one helps to build a reflective organisation. They are:

- *Action pathway: value.* Building a reflective organisation means that a critical mass of staff need to subscribe to the shared value of engaging in collaborative forms of r-learning and doing this in a systematic, supported, rigorous and public manner.

- *Action pathway: conversation.* Building a reflective organisation means that we need to:
    - create the opportunity; and
    - have the ability to use the power of the positive question to strengthen collective capacity and capability to both imagine and build (even) better services for patients/clients.
- *Action pathway: user.* Building a reflective organisation means that we need to sustain conversations of positive regard with service users through:
    - trust
    - engagement
    - open and reflective listening
    - feedback.

    Progress along this action pathway requires us to ask the reflective questions 'What can I learn from service users' experience?', 'How can I respond positively to this' and 'How can learning from service users become an organisation-wide work habit?'
- *Action pathway: leadership.* Building a reflective organisation means that we need to develop a critical mass of staff:
    - with tipping-point leadership skills;
    - who can exercise leadership with an appreciative eye;
    - who can establish and sustain an appreciative disposition across the organisation;
    - who work from the positive present.

    Progress along this action pathway requires us to ask the reflective question 'How can we have more staff who can lead through appreciation?'
- *Action pathway: team.* Building a reflective organisation means that we need to:
    - amplify the number of 'have moments' for staff;
    - nurture the conditions for developing collective wisdom;
    - actively draw upon open-space technology.

A force for change

Finally, I set out a practical force for change, one that helps us build a reflective healthcare organisation. In its totality I called this RAISE. Its components describe five forces that need to operate in order to give us the much needed momentum to progress along one or more action pathways-to-scale. The forces are:

R = *reflecting*
Systematically, rigorously, supportively and publicly learning from reflecting on our practice. The driving force begins with developing positive appreciations. This takes us in the direction of positive action.

A = appreciating

This is a force in two parts: appreciating how people and organisational cultures serve to liberate or constrain us, and appreciating how articulating individual, team and organisational 'best practices' provides a constructive force for creating a positive vision of the future.

I = interacting

This essentially refers to how we can shift away from interacting using re-loading and downloading habits, to interactions that are fuelled by reflective, generative and transformational conversations, or, in a nutshell, more positive and hopeful conversations.

S = strategising

Scaling up r-learning requires a strategy. Strategising refers to the process of strategy formation. The word includes the practices available for shaping it, together with an understanding of the consequences of that shaping.

E = energising

Making progress in building a reflective healthcare organisation requires energy. Energy management and renewal are, therefore, important ways to help make this a healthy pursuit. Reflecting on our energy levels (over- and underuse) is essential because energy (not just time) is essential in building the reflective organisation. Different kinds of energy provide a different force for change.

Towards a full-stop

Building a reflective healthcare organisation is an ambitious undertaking. It may require us to make a significant shift in our thinking and in our relationships with others. It is based on a belief that we *do* have the capability to work together and the capacity to continuously improve services, and that we *can* be caring towards and appreciative of one another, as long as we retain our humanness. As the Zulu word *ubuntu* reminds us, we are only a person through other persons. This book adds to an individualistic reflective practice, a more collective and collegial form. I have called it *reflective learning*. In doing so, I have tried to embrace the fact that we, as individuals, are a part of a greater (inclusive) collective whole. So, building the reflective healthcare organisation may only be achieved with an appreciative social conscience and unity.

I hope you have enjoyed this book. Above all, I hope you have found something useful in it as you contemplate building a reflective healthcare organisation that benefits your patients and clients and supports your staff, so that they can be the best they can.

Index